AGAINST ALL ODDS

A Practical Guide to Successfully Navigate
Psychosis and Behavioral Health Systems

Gary Tsai, M.D.

Foreword by Patrick J. Kennedy,
Former U.S. Representative (D-RI) and
Founder of The Kennedy Forum

AGAINST ALL ODDS: *A Practical Guide to Successfully Navigate Psychosis and Behavioral Health Systems*

www.AgainstAllOddsToday.com

Copyright © 2022 Gary Tsai, M.D.

Paperback ISBN: 979-8-834799-12-2

Publisher
10-10-10 Publishing
Markham, ON   Canada

Printed in the United States of America and Canada

To my mom for teaching me about unconditional love, and my dad for showing me how to be a good father; to my brother for being there for me during our journey, my unimaginably supportive wife, and all those touched by psychosis and other serious behavioral health conditions.

Table of Contents

Foreword

From the first moment I met Dr. Gary Tsai, his passion for behavioral health was clear. His documentary on psychosis, *Voices*; his clinical work as a psychiatrist and addiction physician; and consultations with families across the country have helped thousands of people better understand and seek help for serious mental illness.

Dr. Tsai – a prominent physician executive who is board certified in psychiatry and addiction medicine and responsible for leading the largest substance use system in the country – also happens to be a very skilled communicator with unparalleled knowledge about behavioral health disorders and treatment. His lived experience from growing up with a mother with schizophrenia and his knack for explaining complex issues in simple ways have made him an excellent author.

Against All Odds walks readers through the challenges so many families face in trying to get help for a loved one with serious mental illness—and offers astute insights and tips to successfully navigate these challenges. Through his unique perspective as an expert and as someone who has walked this journey personally, Dr. Tsai illustrates important considerations for all caregivers with grace and compassion. The book is an invaluable tool for laypeople and experienced clinicians alike.

Simply put, I know of no better person to speak on the issue of how to care for a loved one with serious mental illness than Dr. Tsai.

Patrick J. Kennedy
Former U.S. Representative (D-RI)
and Founder of The Kennedy Forum

Acknowledgments

Sincere gratitude to all my current and former colleagues and patients, particularly from my time at the University of California at Davis, San Mateo, San Diego, and Los Angeles, for broadening my knowledge and perspectives.

To my family and friends, thank you for being there for me during the good times and bad.

I also want to thank those on the frontlines supporting clients and families impacted by serious mental illness every day, working tirelessly to improve access and address inequities for people living with behavioral health conditions, including:

- Behavioral health practitioners and community-based organizations serving our communities on the ground
- National Alliance on Mental Illness (NAMI)
- Treatment Advocacy Center
- National Council
- American Psychiatric Association
- American Society of Addiction Medicine
- National Association of Social Workers
- American Psychological Association
- American Association for Marriage and Family Therapy
- National Association for Addiction Professionals
- The Kennedy Forum
- One Mind

- Strong365

... And countless others whose work inspires and moves the behavioral health needle forward.

Chapter One

Introduction

Serious mental illnesses, or SMI, are behavioral health (mental health and substance use) conditions that result in significant functional impairment. They include conditions such as schizophrenia, schizo-affective disorder, and bipolar disorder.

A common hallmark of serious mental illness and a particular focus of this book is psychosis, which is characterized by a state of discon-nection from reality and altered auditory and visual perceptions, thought processes, and movements. Individuals experiencing psychosis will often hear voices (auditory hallucinations), see things that others do not (visual hallucinations), feel paranoid about the well-being of themselves or loved ones, and/or present with disorganized behaviors.

The emergence of serious mental illness and psychosis is often a defining moment in the lives of those impacted.

That was certainly the case when my mom began hearing derogatory voices in the form of auditory hallucinations. We now know she was exhibiting the early signs of paranoid schizophrenia. But when you are ten years old and your mother suddenly asks why you felt she was a bad mother, surprise and confusion is your initial reaction.

I had no idea what spurred this question but was in the middle of playing with my brother and didn't give the question a second thought. I said, *"Of course not!"* and turned back to my brother, wiping the sweat from my brow before throwing him the football.

A few days later, she asked me the same question again. Now I sensed something was wrong. When I told my dad, he initially downplayed the encounter as a miscommunication.

Years later, he told me that he had been noticing increasingly concerning symptoms for years but did his best to shield us from worry about my mom's condition.

My father explained that the truth was that my biochemist mother with a Ph.D. was hearing voices and displaying the telltale signs of paranoid schizophrenia. This was the same person who lovingly ate leftovers so her family could enjoy her freshly cooked beef and broccoli; the loving mother that would drop everything to help her kids with their homework and last-minute school projects.

Our mom transformed into an increasingly unpredictable, angry person who was disconnected from reality. Evenings often consisted of her yelling at the television, her eyes filled with rage as she responded to the relentless, paranoid delusions and hallucinations that plagued her mind. During the day, she would fight with my dad and accuse him of infidelity or working with spies trying to undermine her.

Since the brain naturally tends to focus on familiar things, many people who have psychosis hear voices and have paranoid thoughts or delusions centered around who and what they know best. This was the case with my mom. Her voices and delusions revolved around those closest to her, principally her family, and the themes that hit at the heart of her greatest worries.

As a result, she would hear things that validated her greatest fears: voices telling her she was an inadequate mother, that my father was unfaithful in their marriage, or voices from strangers saying that my brother and I would not be successful because we played too much and needed to study more. Paranoid schizophrenia made all of my mom's deepest and darkest fears and insecurities materialize around her.

As her son and caregiver, being relegated to a powerless bystander was simultaneously heartbreaking and frustrating.

Although she would get angry and scary at times, she was also simultaneously kind, gentle, and loving during periods when her symptoms relented. But as the years went by, her disease progressed. Periods of clarity and calm became less frequent.

This led to calls to the police from neighbors and repeated visits to the emergency room. These encounters often resulted in brief episodes of treatment, but no ongoing care.

We struggled to convince her to accept help. There were countless attempts to rationalize with her, explaining that it did not make sense why the government would want to track our activities. We pointed out that we couldn't say derogatory things about her when we were not at home. We even tried recording our conversations throughout the day to prove to her that the things she was hearing were not actually said. None of this worked.

During one of my attempts to convince her to accept help, I asked her to consider the possibility that the voices she was hearing were, in fact, her brain playing tricks on her. Without pause, she responded, *"I never make up what I hear!"*

In her fervent and unwavering refusals to accept treatment, it was clear that more than simple psychological denial, my mom genuinely did not believe that she had a problem.

Frustration and desperation began to mount. We saw her gradually lose her personal relationships, her career as a cancer research scientist, and eventually, connections with the world outside of our immediate family.

The fact that we were all she had left strengthened our bond and desire to stand by her side. But we were also human throughout each painful episode. We got upset when she continued to decline care despite her obvious need, and embarrassed when she got upset due to her paranoid delusions in public. But there were also happy times when we were a typical family enjoying a trip to the mall or a vacation at the beach. Only much later did I realize how important it was that my mother knew she was loved throughout these ups and downs.

Decades passed before my mother received the help she needed. It was ultimately not by her choice either. Eventually, hallucinating and causing a scene at a post office led to a week-long disappearance at the local jail and a trespassing charge—a classic case of the criminalization of mental illness. This episode then resulted in her being admitted into a court-ordered outpatient treatment program.

When she entered this program, she was finally able to receive the ongoing treatment and care that she had needed for years. By this time, I was a freshly minted psychiatrist and was as prepared as one could possibly be to navigate the complexities of our behavioral health system. I embedded myself into my mother's care, regularly connecting with her psychiatrist along with the other professionals on her care team.

For the first time ever, her treatment stuck.

Our phone conversations were the clearest examples of her recovery. No longer did calls end with paranoid accusations. Instead, she talked about her day and asked me how my work was going. After 25 years, I was having amazingly rich and meaningful conversations with my mom and getting to know her in an entirely new and different way.

That said, even when she was stable in her recovery, my mother was never fully aware of her schizophrenia. If you asked her why she took her antipsychotic medication, she would say it helped her sleep. Deep down, I suspect she may have noticed that the medications quieted the world around her. The whispers and chatter that were generally at the forefront of her mind seemed to get quieter and move to the background, at times barely perceptible.

As my mother grew older, her psychosis also evolved. It dwelled less on dark and painful thoughts and focused more on benign subjects, like the time I came home to a massive value pack of blueberry scones she had bought because her voices told her I wanted them. In reality, I think the seed of that hallucination originated from her reluctance to spend money on these types of guilty pleasures for herself.

Because my mom believed her hallucinations were real, she never believed she heard voices. Therein lies the tightrope of trying to treat someone with serious mental illness who does not have insight or self-awareness of their condition. In these instances, obtaining care is inevitably an uphill battle.

Despite how pivotal and relatively common serious mental illness is, seeking help in these situations remains variable and unclear at best, and inhumane at worst. Regardless of one's background or available resources, navigating care for a loved one in this situation can be extraordinarily draining, confusing, and lonely.

Through the lens of a psychiatrist that grew up with a mother with schizophrenia, and whose family struggled for over two decades to get her care, the purpose of this book is to make the process of navigating behavioral health systems easier by empowering readers with the perspective gained by someone who has gone through it, both personally and professionally.

By providing a deeper understanding of serious mental illness and how to approach individuals with these conditions, options for care, and sharing perspectives from a behavioral health expert with firsthand experience as a family member of someone with serious mental illness, this practical guide unpacks some of the most common pitfalls confronted when navigating the complexity of behavioral health care.

Chapter Two

The Basics – What, When, & Why

Serious mental illnesses affect approximately 5% of the general population. While this represents a relatively small minority when compared with the broader population, this still means that there are over 13 million people in the United States who are impacted, as well as their extended network of family and friends.

Its human, societal, and economic impact is sizable in terms of suffering, premature death, suicides, avoidable hospitalizations, preventable incarcerations, and other poor outcomes.

Bipolar disorder is the most prevalent serious mental illness, affecting about 2–3% of the U.S. population. This is followed by schizophrenia (~1% prevalence) and schizoaffective disorder (<1% prevalence). Serious mental illness can also include people with co-occurring substance use. In these cases, signs and symptoms of serious mental illness may fluctuate depending on the frequency of substance use, including but not limited to methamphetamine and cannabis.

What to Look For

In healthcare, **signs** are things that can be observed, and **symptoms** are experiences described by patients.

Examples of <u>signs</u> include:
· Blood pressure

- Coughing
- Someone speaking to themselves

Examples of <u>symptoms</u> include:
- Stomach aches
- Fatigue
- Depression

The signs and symptoms of serious mental illness generally become apparent between adolescence and adulthood. Although they can present outside of these time windows, such as during childhood or late adulthood, most signs and symptoms are evident by age 30.

Some of the most common initial presentations of serious mental illness include:
- Sleep and appetite changes
- Declining function or participation in school, work, or social activities
- Withdrawal from social and recreational activities
- Changes in mood
- Decline in personal hygiene
- Problems with concentrating/focusing
- Unusual thought patterns and/or logic
- Atypical attributions of meanings or beliefs
- Uncharacteristic behaviors

Most of the time, these signs and symptoms have psychiatric origins. However, there are also atypical causes of serious mental illness that are not rooted in a psychiatric condition, such as tumors, infections, electrolyte or hormonal imbalances, or other medical conditions. Unique presentations—such as signs and symptoms that are unconventional in characteristic or timing—often warrant a thorough medical workup for alternative explanations.

In these cases, lab tests may be necessary to rule out non-psychiatric causes of the symptoms. Head imaging (e.g., MRI or CT scans) can also be helpful when there are co-occurring neurological symptoms, or another rationale for ruling out structural deficiencies such as a tumor causing dysfunction in particular brain regions, which may result in psychotic symptoms, for example. That said, this is not necessary in most cases, as psychiatric conditions and/or substance use explain the majority of symptoms suggestive of serious mental illness. It is important to note that for someone to be accurately diagnosed, their signs and symptoms must not be explained by substance use.

Schizophrenia

Schizophrenia is a psychiatric condition typically associated with psychosis. Positive symptoms of schizophrenia can be thought of as experiences that are additive that should not be there, such as auditory hallucinations, visual hallucinations, or paranoia. Alternatively, negative symptoms of schizophrenia can be equated to qualities that are typically apparent but absent, such as a lack of interest or motivation, an inability to express or feel pleasure, decreased speech, decreased social engagement, and reductions in purposeful activity. Disorganization is another hallmark of schizophrenia.

The collective impact of these symptoms, which can be present in any combination, can lead to problems maintaining hygiene, thinking clearly or rationally, and an inability to engage with others. In about 10% of cases of schizophrenia, psychosis can result in a state of catatonia, resulting in a person exhibiting immobility, abnormal movements, an inability to speak, or mimicking others' actions or speech.

It is important to note that despite depictions in popular culture that often confuse the two, split or multiple personalities are not the same as schizophrenia and are instead known as dissociative identity disorders. These are complex psychological conditions where individuals present with at least two distinct personality states and cases are often associated with severe trauma. Dissociative identity disorders are distinctly different from schizophrenia and do not indicate a psychotic process.

Schizoaffective Disorder

Schizoaffective disorders are primary psychotic conditions with secondary mood (manic or depressive) disorders. A key characteristic that differentiates schizoaffective disorder from schizophrenia is that mood symptoms are more prominent with the former compared to the latter. Similarly, schizoaffective disorder is different than mood disorders with psychotic features because psychotic symptoms are more prominent with schizoaffective disorder and may be apparent without any manic or depressive episodes for periods of time of at least two weeks.

Bipolar Disorder

Bipolar disorder is a severe mood disorder characterized by fluctuations between "highs" known as mania, and "lows" in the form of depression. Manic episodes of bipolar disorder are often associated with poor sleep, increased energy and activity, racing thoughts, rapid speech, an elevated sense of self-importance (grandiosity), reckless behavior, and symptoms of psychosis. Alternatively, depressive episodes of bipolar disorder are defined by feelings of emptiness, sadness, worthlessness, a lack of interest in activities, and the inability to experience joy.

There are two types of bipolar disorder: Type I and Type II. Type I is more severe and characterized by full manic episodes. Type II is associated with less intense "highs" known as hypomanic episodes.

Co-Occurring Serious Mental Illness and Substance Use

Individuals with serious mental illness may also have co-occurring substance use disorders. Given that substance use can lead to psychotic or mood symptoms, and vice versa, the challenge with these cases is determining whether the symptoms of serious mental illness came first or the substance use.

But regardless of the order and what happened first, the ideal approach to treating someone with co-occurring serious mental illness and substance use is to treat the conditions simultaneously. Given that accessing care for substance use presents its own set of challenges and those that confront those with serious mental illness, finding programs offering treatment services for individuals with co-occurring disorders can be challenging. For this reason, if one cannot find a program specializing in care for people with co-occurring disorders, it is sometimes necessary to have someone receive their mental health services in one setting while receiving their substance use services in another.

Course of Condition

It is important to recognize that recovery looks different for everyone, both in terms of the journey and the end outcome of what recovery looks like. While some individuals with serious mental illness exhibit time-limited symptoms and recover after only one or two episodes of symptoms, most cases follow a chronic and relapsing course with fluctuating symptoms and functioning over a longer period. Various factors significantly influence the course of one's condition, such as:

- Self-awareness
- Responsiveness to medications
- Support networks
- Social determinants of health (e.g., housing, social connectedness, etc.)

As is often the case with complex health conditions, there is no silver bullet to guarantee recovery. There are only treatments and strategies to increase the likelihood of recovery in its various forms. For some people with serious mental illness, recovery means being able to independently get groceries and prepare meals, whereas for others, it means finishing graduate school and being offered one's dream job. In all instances, support for both the individual suffering from the condition and their caregiver(s) is essential.

Anosognosia

Approximately 40–50% of individuals with serious mental illness live with a condition called anosognosia. Anosognosia results from damage to the areas of the brain responsible for self-awareness and self-reflection. Unlike typical denial, which is psychological in origin, the cause of anosognosia is anatomical in the brain. In these instances, people with anosognosia are neurobiologically unable to realize that they have a psychiatric condition.

Given that one of the fundamental prerequisites of seeking help is self-awareness, anosognosia presents incredible challenges for those suffering from serious mental illness since most mental health systems are designed for people seeking care voluntarily. Unfortunately, even with intense engagement strategies for those with anosognosia, involuntary or court-mandated care is sometimes required to facilitate access to the care they need to avoid tragedies such as imprisonment, homelessness, or premature death.

Theories of the Causes of Schizophrenia

The causes of mental health conditions are multi-dimensional and generally cannot be explained by a single root cause. But there are several theories regarding the origins of serious mental illness that revolve around a combination of nature (genetics) and nurture (environmental factors). Given that literature regarding the contributing causes of schizophrenia is arguably the most established of all serious mental illness, this section will focus on schizophrenia.

Most genetic theories of schizophrenia assume that the condition is not caused by genes alone, but rather by a combination of genes in the presence of environmental factors such as trauma or certain infections that may make someone more susceptible to developing schizophrenia. Twin studies of schizophrenia have suggested concordance rates of 30–60%, meaning that even with identical twins that share the same genetics, the likelihood of both twins developing schizophrenia is only 30–60%. This supports the notion that genetics alone cannot fully explain the heritability of schizophrenia.

While the prevalence of schizophrenia is 1% in the general population, being a first-degree relative of someone with schizophrenia comes with a 10% increased risk of developing schizophrenia. Although the percentages cited here convey an impression of definitiveness, the reality is that the genetics of schizophrenia and other serious mental illnesses are extraordinarily complex, and much is still unknown about the origins of these conditions.

In addition to the genetic theory of schizophrenia, neurochemical theories of schizophrenia are also popular. Neurotransmitters such as dopamine, glutamate, and gamma-aminobutyric acid (GABA) are chemicals that carry messages between brain cells known as neurons. Various neurotransmitters interact with one another in different areas of the brain in highly complex ways. While increased dopamine and reduced glutamate and GABA in some regions of the brain are associated with psychotic symptoms, it is unclear whether these neurotransmitter patterns are causes or effects of schizophrenia.

The developmental theory of schizophrenia focuses on disruptions during the brain's intricate development process from the fetal period into adulthood. With this theory, the focus is less on what causes the disruption and more on the fact that any interference (e.g., maternal illness during the fetal period, chemicals such as drugs or medications, malnutrition, trauma, or extreme stress) during critical periods of brain development may lead to dysfunctional brain processes later in life.

Another similar theory of schizophrenia focuses on infectious agents, inflammation, and the immune system, all of which are related. For example, there is evidence that some individuals with schizophrenia have high levels of inflammation in their bodies, with antibodies to certain viruses or parasites that indicate prior infections. The interactions between bacteria, viruses, and other pathogens in the gut microbiome have also been theorized to be potentially related to conditions such as schizophrenia.

Since schizophrenia, schizoaffective disorder, and bipolar disorder are more practically seen as a diagnostic spectrum as opposed to three distinct conditions, there are likely shared causes across these conditions. Many of the theories described above regarding the cause(s) of schizophrenia are mutually inclusive, and most likely, the root causes of the condition involve several different factors.

Chapter Three

How to Approach a Loved One with Serious Mental Illness (While Taking Care of Yourself!)

To address and cope with psychosis and serious mental illness, one must understand both the condition as well as the programs and system within which it is treated. The deepest understanding is attained when "textbook" comprehension is combined with knowledge acquired through lived experience—when you are affected personally or experience it by proxy via a friend or family member.

With decades of experience as a family member of a loved one with schizophrenia, and as a psychiatrist, this chapter consolidates my personal and professional experiences related to two of the most challenging aspects of managing serious mental illnesses: 1) engaging loved ones and overcoming resistance to treatment; and 2) self-care.

It is important to understand what someone with psychosis is experiencing in order to develop effective approaches to engage them.

Let's start with the basics—namely, the brain. It is our command center. Our brain tells us how to think, feel, and behave. It is the primary way we perceive the world via our five basic senses: sound, sight, smell, touch, and taste. In short, our brain determines our reality.

In most cases, the reality constructed by our brain is consistent with the reality of others around us, and there is shared agreement about that reality. In the case of a brain experiencing psychosis, this reality is distorted due to misfiring from some of the billions of brain cells, called neurons, connected to one another via trillions of synapses in the brain. These synaptic connections between neurons form brain pathways that govern overall brain activity. Certain damaged brain pathways are more relevant to psychosis than others.

If one thinks of the brain as the engine of a car, this particular car engine is extraordinarily complex with a plethora of moving parts. With more parts, there are also more opportunities for things to go wrong. The brain typically undergoes a process of self-maintenance called synaptic pruning to get rid of unnecessary neurons and preserve those needed for brain pathways that serve critical functions. However, this pruning process can go awry and either get rid of neuronal connections that are important to keep, or maintain things that should be removed. It has been suggested that errors in synaptic pruning may contribute to schizophrenia risk.

Usually, when someone hears a bird chirping, their ears pick up the sound and transmit it to their brains. This activates the auditory pathways of the brain to let the person know that they are hearing something. When someone with schizophrenia experiences auditory hallucinations and hears voices that others cannot hear, the brain's auditory center responsible for hearing is misfiring and inappropriately activated in the absence of sound. This results in the individual hearing something because their brain tells them they're hearing something, even though there is no external stimulus. This has been validated by imaging studies of the brain that show the auditory centers being activated while someone is hallucinating, even though there was no external stimulus. This is why auditory hallucinations are so real to the people experiencing them and are not "made up"—because their brain is undergoing the same process as what happens when there is an external noise.

Delusions are fixed beliefs that are often based on hallucinations or misinterpreted cues related to psychosis. They are not based on generally accepted reality. With paranoia and delusions, the brain inappropriately associates what typically would be benign stimuli with activation of the areas of the brain responsible for fear, anxiety, and other functions involved in paranoia.

Similar to hallucinations, individuals with paranoia and delusions cannot control the way their brain interprets these stimuli. To them, these experiences are as real as how we would feel if a shadowy, menacing figure followed us into a dark alley.

There is another aspect of psychosis that is far more sinister. For many people with these symptoms, the hallucinations, paranoia, and delusions that underly their psychosis represent their deepest, darkest fears. For example, a doctor who has trained much of their life to do their job competently may hallucinate or have delusions revolving around their clinical aptitude. Similarly, new mothers may suffer from hallucinations or delusions that relate to the safety of their children or their capabilities caring for them.

The reason for this common phenomenon is because, at its most fundamental level, the brain is a complex web of pathways and networks whose primary job is to make sense of the world through connections and associations. It is also connected to one's feelings, emotions, psychology, and physical body. Since someone's most common anxieties or worries often result in the brain areas responsible for these feelings being activated more often than other less used areas, these conscious and subconscious tendencies tend to be common areas of focus for the brain. Thus, symptoms of psychosis naturally have an increased likelihood of focusing on the things that are most salient and familiar to that particular brain.

Another similar and unfortunate aspect of psychotic symptoms is the tendency for them to be directed at loved ones. Given how deeply memories of loved ones are stored in our brain, the brain is naturally wired to make associations between those we care about and our experiences and feelings. While some psychosis is focused on strangers, most often, the delusions and hallucinations that individuals experience are centered around family, friends, and those they care about the most, because that is what is more familiar and accessible to the brain.

Psychotic symptoms are also responsive to societal factors of the times. For example, while individuals with psychosis today may feel paranoid about being tracked by computer chips implanted in their bodies, those with paranoia during the pre-computer age were more likely to focus on being tracked by spies or other technology appropriate for the time.

As noted in Chapter Two, anosognosia is an additional complexity of serious mental illnesses that accompanies upwards of half of individuals with these conditions. This limits the insight and ability for one to self-reflect on symptoms and apply reason in a way that facilitates help-seeking. With impaired self-awareness, it is nearly impossible for people with anosognosia to recognize and accept their psychotic symptoms as something that requires treatment, given the absence of the necessary precursor of self-recognition.

Considering all the above, living with and caring for someone with serious mental illness can span the full spectrum of emotions. Bad days where symptoms are particularly pronounced can be immensely frustrating and deflating. Good days where you're able to effectively communicate and connect with your loved one can be joyful and feel as if an extraordinary weight has been lifted from your shoulders.

As a result, living with serious mental illness or caring for someone with these conditions can accurately be described as a roller coaster. An integral element of maximizing the likelihood of a positive outcome in these situations is having compassion and empathy, not just for the person with the condition, but also for yourself and the circle of involved caregivers. Caregiving can be extraordinarily difficult and, to be sustainable, caregivers often need to give themselves a break, both literally and figuratively.

Given the complexity of serious mental illnesses and the intricacies of accessing care, a single intervention or strategy is rarely effective. Effective interventions often require multiple approaches that work synergistically with one another to increase the likelihood of a positive outcome.

With this in mind, two critical focus areas to optimize outcomes for individuals with serious mental illness are:

- Effective approaches to treat and support impacted individuals and caregivers (Chapter Three); and
- Knowledge about behavioral health systems, programs, laws, practitioners, and payers to facilitate successful navigation of these complex components of seeking care (Chapter Four).

One of the primary challenges to getting help for someone with serious mental illness is often convincing them that they need help in the first place. Even if it is clear to everyone around them, whether due to anosognosia, denial, or other reasons, individuals with serious mental illness do not always accept or recognize they need help. Usually, this resistance may manifest in the form of an individual declining treatment, refusing to engage in helpful activities, or may even come from family members that struggle to accept that their loved might have a psychiatric condition. In these instances, the resistance and accompanying emotions of trying to manage that resistance go hand in hand. Learning to recognize that association and implementing strategies to address them is critical.

Principles of motivational interviewing are one of the most practical approaches to dealing with resistance that anyone can learn. Motivational interviewing is a method of communication that facilitates behavior change by actively guiding discussions and having others identify their own meaning and intrinsic desire for change, as opposed to directly confronting their resistance. The main reason for avoiding direct confrontation of resistance is because it rarely works.

Put yourself in the position of a person with paranoid schizophrenia that is hearing voices telling you that your friends and family are trying to undermine you by telling you that you need psychiatric help. The medicine they suggest you take is both unnecessary and comes with side effects. Also, assume that you have anosognosia and cannot self-reflect on your condition. In this situation, simply having your parents tell you that you need help is unlikely to sway you, as it contradicts your experience of reality.

A motivational interviewing approach to the above example of paranoid schizophrenia would involve learning more about why that person thinks that others are trying to undermine them, what they think about medications, any positive or negative experiences they have had with it, as well as what things or situations in their life they would like to see improved. This allows you to explore opportunities to align treatment with a client's priorities and beliefs. For example, one may indicate that their sleep is being disrupted at night because their neighbors are making derogatory statements to them through the walls. In this instance, a motivational interviewing approach might focus on the impact of medications to improve sleep. While the antipsychotic medication may be primarily working to minimize the hallucinations leading to the disrupted sleep, the secondary benefit is improved sleep, and thus focusing the individual on this desired outcome may help to address this resistance and create more openness to trying this intervention.

A fundamental aim of motivational interviewing is finding the most effective strategy to facilitate behavioral change. It is important to recognize that while one can't always debunk a firmly held belief, one can validate the emotion behind that belief. It can be incredibly beneficial to identify points of agreement, even amid significant disagreement on core issues, such as whether someone needs help. This is particularly important in situations of anosognosia, where an individual is unable to self-reflect on their condition. In these situations, they feel all the emotions associated with these frightening experiences, even if they are not based on the reality of those around them.

In sum, motivational interviewing should be thought of more as a non-judgmental style of communicating that many people utilize in some form every day already. It can be used for all sorts of behavior change, from encouraging someone to change their diet or exercise more, to getting your child to do their homework. Instead of giving advice or persuading, motivational interviewing uses curiosity to overcome ambivalence. Although motivational interviewing is unlikely to be the silver bullet to convince everyone with serious mental illness and anosognosia to accept care if they firmly do not believe they need it, it can be a helpful tool to sow seeds of change.

In addition to employing strategies to address resistance, caregivers also need to cope with the emotions commonly associated with these challenges. Trying to convince someone to do something they do not want to do, on a regular basis, is emotionally and physically draining. Feelings of anger and frustration are very natural and common reactions in these situations. Learning how to recognize, accept, and productively deal with these emotions will benefit both the person who needs help and caregivers.

There are several strategies that may be helpful in these situations:

- The brain has difficulty feeling two strong emotions simultaneously, so engaging in activities that induce positive emotions when one feels angry can quell destructive anger.
- Anger tends to lead to rumination about whatever incited the anger, so breaking rumination cycles with distractions can be highly effective.
- While venting and blowing off steam works when done constructively, such as venting to a spouse or friend, destructive venting can serve as practicing how to be angry and *"strengthen your anger muscle."*

We often think, say, or do things when we're angry that may feel good in the moment, but do not feel good after we've calmed down. This can be one way to differentiate between *constructive* and *destructive* venting. *Constructive* venting often results in someone feeling better, not immediately after but 10 minutes after they calm down. In contrast, *destructive* venting makes one feel worse even after they calm down. Engaging in *constructive* venting is helpful, whereas surrendering to *destructive* venting is not.

The latter portion of this chapter is focused on compassion fatigue. Compassion fatigue is generally identified by feelings of anger or guilt toward the affected individual or caregivers, including yourself. Given the intensity and emotions often involved in caring for someone with serious mental illness, compassion fatigue is a nearly universal struggle. One of the most fundamental ways to prevent and manage compassion fatigue is to have a realistic sense of what is and is not under your control, and recognizing that it is often best to focus on what is under your control, given that trying to control things that are not under your control may be futile.

To this aim, one of the only things we can control is ourselves—how we think, what we do, and at times how we feel. There are many aspects of caring for someone that are not directly under our control—federal, state, and local policies regarding care, legal barriers, the quality of staff at treatment sites, whether a loved one responds to medications, how other people respond to our loved ones with serious mental illness, etc. While we may advocate and do other things to increase the likelihood that things will go well, we must recognize that all we can do is our best.

Another point of stress is someone's persistent delusions. Sometimes these delusions are paranoid (i.e., people are following and trying to harm me) or grandiose (i.e., the president of the United States desperately needs my help, so I need to reach out).

Regardless of the focus of the delusions, it's essential to realize that delusions are seeds that have already been planted by psychosis. While treating psychosis can reduce future delusions, it often doesn't undo or remove the seed of ideas and delusions already in place. For example, if someone with chronic delusions were effectively treated, the generation of future delusions would be limited, but their delusions before treatment would likely remain in some form. For this reason, just because someone continues to have delusions does not necessarily mean that they are actively psychotic. This is an important distinction because using delusions as a marker of treatment progress often causes unnecessary discouragement, when the reality is that someone who is psychotic may be getting better even if they continue to express old delusions.

Adequately tending to your needs as a caregiver is one of the most critical components of caring for someone with serious mental illness. Giving oneself enough autonomy and space to maintain a sense of self is essential. Whether it's a weekly basketball game you play with your friends, a standing dinner date you have with your partner, or something as simple as being able to catch up on your favorite TV show, the ability to continue to engage in activities that are important to you is a foundational requirement of sustainable caregiving.

Chapter Four

Overview of Behavioral Health Systems, Laws, Practitioners, and Insurance Types

In physics and thermodynamics, the entropy principle states that the spontaneous evolution of systems is more likely to result in disorder and complexity over time than it is to become simpler and more ordered. This is also true for behavioral health systems, which are generally more accurately described as haphazardly constructed as opposed to thoughtfully designed. A key reason for this is because as opportunities for new programs, priorities, funding, and laws arise, the path of least resistance is inevitably to take an additive approach to the pre-existing system as opposed to a synergizing approach that wholly deconstructs the system and redesigns it with the new components in mind. In this case, the inertia of behavioral health systems moves toward complexity, and it takes more work to simplify processes than it does to complicate them.

While this chapter will not re-design behavioral health systems, it will fast-track the process of learning about the various components of these systems to enhance understanding and make them easier to navigate.

Although behavioral health systems, policies, and laws differ in jurisdictions across the country, some commonalities are generally consistent throughout. This chapter focuses on better understanding four key essentials of successful care:

- The various types of services and treatment settings that comprise behavioral health systems

- Behavioral health laws
- Types of behavioral health practitioners
- Different payers and insurance for these services

Behavioral Health Systems

One of the most challenging aspects of navigating behavioral health systems is understanding the different levels of care and types of services that are typically available. The graphic below organizes behavioral health systems into several fundamental settings:

- Crisis response
- Emergency services
- Acute settings
- Inpatient or hospital-based care
- Sub-acute settings (e.g., residential non-hospital-based settings)
- Outpatient settings in the community

Overview of Behavioral Health Settings

Level 0

Crisis Response
- Mobile Crisis Intervention Teams (CIT)
- Law Enforcement

Level 1

Emergency
- Typical emergency room in general acute hospital vs. Psychiatric Emergency Room

Level 2

Acute (Inpatient/Hospital-Based Settings)
- Psychiatric Hospitals
- State Hospitals (forensics)
- Inpatient substance use disorder treatment and withdrawal management

Level 3

Sub-Acute (Residential & Non-Hospital-Based Settings)
- Locked Residential (licensed as Mental Health Rehabilitation Center, Skilled Nursing Facility [SNF] / Special Treatment Program [STP])
- Unlocked Residential
- Enriched Residential Services (housing + intensive behavioral health services)
- Residential substance use disorder treatment (various intensity levels) and withdrawal management

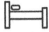

Level 4

Outpatient (Clinic or Community-Based Settings)
- Full Service Partnership (FSP) or Assertive Community Treatment (ACT) teams
- Outpatient mental health services + Board and Care / other housing options
- Different types of outpatient substance use disorder treatment and withdrawal management (e.g., outpatient, intensive outpatient, Opioid Treatment Programs)

The type of setting that someone is best served in depends on a combination of the severity and acuity of their condition, the types of services available in a community, and the capacity of those services to meet the needs of the specific individual in question.

Just because someone has a severe diagnosis does not mean that they are acute or need to be hospitalized. This is because someone with a serious diagnosis could also be stable in terms of their baseline symptoms. For example, while someone with chronic paranoid schizophrenia is generally considered to have a *severe* psychiatric condition, they are not regarded as *acute* unless their condition is unstable and needs care at a higher level of care. Someone with chronic psychotic symptoms, despite receiving treatment, may be considered stable and non-acute even if they continue to have symptoms, the same way that someone with diabetes may be considered stable and non-acute even if they have higher than normal blood sugar levels.

Alternatively, an unstable and acute person with schizophrenia would be actively experiencing distressing psychotic symptoms that are worse than their baseline level of functioning. On the other hand, someone may have a psychiatric condition that is typically considered relatively benign, such as social anxiety, but the situation can become unstable, acute, and require hospitalization, for example if the individual becomes suicidal because of an exacerbation of their anxiety.

When placing people into specific behavioral health settings, the goal is to match individualized needs with the setting of care that best approximates those needs. Levels of care that are matched accurately with client needs have generally shown to result in better outcomes than placing clients into either a higher level of care that is more restrictive than they need, or a lower level or care that inadequately addresses the level of psychiatric acuity that someone exhibits. Unfortunately, capacity limitations far too often prevent access to needed services in behavioral health systems. As a result, matching available mental health and substance use services with individual client needs is often more challenging than one would anticipate.

Crisis Response

Crisis care for mental health and substance use conditions involves de-escalating and triaging crises such as suicidality or escalating behaviors associated with acute psychosis, often in the field. While this is not always the case, behavioral health crisis response teams often can place legal holds (up to 72 hours in most jurisdictions) on individuals to compel further psychiatric evaluation as needed.

There are typically two types of behavioral health crisis response. The first is where first responders (e.g., law enforcement, fire departments) are the primary responders, while the second incorporates mental health professionals in the process. The latter sometimes goes by different program names but may be called Crisis Intervention Teams (CIT) or Psychiatric Emergency Teams (PET). The key characteristic of these programs is that they include behavioral health professionals, such as social workers, psychologists, or peer specialists to help respond to the individual in crisis.

In some models, behavioral health professionals are paired with law enforcement entities when people call 911. Other times, there are specific phone numbers one must contact to connect with local crisis response programs that include behavioral health professionals. It is helpful to determine what programs are available in your area so that you're prepared in the event crisis services are needed in the future.

In calls with emergency responders regarding behavioral health crises, it is helpful to clearly explain the situation, including the following details:

- The reason(s) for and location of your call
- The relationship between the caller and the person who is the focus of the call
- How the individual in question is behaving

- Why you think they're behaving this way
- If they have any behavioral health or medical conditions
- How emergent the situation is and why, including if any weapons are involved or other safety considerations first responders need to be mindful of
- If anything has helped to effectively address similar presentations in the past

The goal is to be as concise and descriptive as possible to provide the responding entity a sense of the situation to start formulating a plan for how to effectively respond. This will maximize the potential for a positive outcome by lessening the likelihood that they are surprised on arrival and giving them time to strategize on their response enroute.

After assessing and de-escalating the situation as needed, the critical decision point for crisis response teams is whether someone needs immediate psychiatric care (e.g., through transportation to an emergency room) or is safe to follow up with behavioral health services in an outpatient (clinic-based) setting. If the former is needed, crisis response teams capable of placing psychiatric holds may execute these holds in the field to facilitate ongoing care in emergency and hospital-based settings. The crisis response process usually lasts up to several hours.

The determination around whether a psychiatric hold is needed is often a legal decision as opposed to a clinical decision involving subjective determinations about dangerousness (i.e., the potential for imminent harm to self or others) or grave disability (i.e., the ability to care for oneself and provide for one's food, shelter, and clothing). Psychiatry is one of the few medical professions to have clinical care so heavily influenced by legal standards and requirements. This is one of the reasons why effective advocacy for a loved one with behavioral health conditions often requires at least a basic understanding of the laws and regulations that govern care.

Generally, outcomes are better when behavioral health professionals are involved in the response to behavioral health crises. If your community offers this option, it is preferable compared to a law enforcement driven response, given the greater familiarity of behavioral health professionals with de-escalation techniques and effective strategies to address individuals in crisis. Unfortunately, there have been increasingly publicized cases of law enforcement responding to behavioral health crises that end with the individual in question getting injured or killed. While people with acute psychiatric presentations do at times become angry, loud, threatening, or even aggressive— particularly when responding to their paranoia or hallucinations—this is the minority of cases as opposed to the majority. Experienced behavioral health professionals are often able to address these situations without force.

Emergency Psychiatric Care

Similar yet distinct from crisis care, psychiatric emergency care usually occurs in an emergency room within a general acute hospital, or an emergency room specifically designed to care for people with psychiatric conditions. Emergency rooms within general acute hospitals are more common. They are the type of hospital that most people imagine and are familiar with in terms of the standard emergency room (e.g., gurneys, smaller rooms sometimes separated by curtains, emergency room doctors, and nurses that use specialized equipment to address emergency conditions, etc.).

Alternatively, psychiatric emergency rooms—sometimes called "Psychiatric Emergency Services (PES)" or "Emergency Psychiatric Units (EPU)"—focus specifically on psychiatric emergencies. These emergency rooms have psychiatrists, nurses, social workers, and peer specialists trained to address psychiatric emergencies. They usually have rooms with furniture, fixings, and equipment used in psychiatric settings to ensure safety.

In general emergency rooms and psychiatric emergency room settings, psychiatric emergencies are triaged to determine the most appropriate treatment and response. Psychiatric care in the emergency setting often involves obtaining a thorough history from the patient and other collateral sources (friends or family), medications to immediately stabilize mental health and substance use symptoms such as severe psychotic, mood, anxiety, and withdrawal symptoms, and assessments to determine the best next steps.

Individuals are typically evaluated in emergency settings for hours up to several days, largely dependent on the severity level of someone's presentation and the availability of care after the emergency setting.

The emergency room assessment generally results in the decision to either admit someone into an acute psychiatric treatment setting if ongoing care is immediately needed, or discharge the patient back into the community, often with a referral for outpatient follow-up.

Given how vital the disposition decision from the emergency setting is, it is generally helpful to contact the emergency room to speak with the psychiatrist or treating physician caring for your loved one. This communication should convey important historical and collateral information about the individual with serious mental illness to ensure that the treating team in the emergency room has the information they need to make informed clinical and legal decisions about the need for ongoing care. Individuals may be symptomatic at home but reconstitute in a more structured setting, such as during an interview with a psychiatrist. In these cases, collateral information from family or friends is vital to ensure that the treating provider has the full clinical perspective to make informed determinations.

The Health Insurance Portability and Accountability Act (HIPAA) is a common challenge in emergency settings, as HIPAA is often cited as the reason why the emergency room cannot verify whether your loved one is there. In these cases, it is important to note that HIPAA governs disclosures of health information from the treating entity to others, but it does not prevent caregivers from providing information to the treating entity. Even if the emergency room cannot verify if your loved one with serious mental illness is a patient, you may explain that HIPPA still allows you to provide critical care information to them in the event they are there. See the *Legalities of Behavioral Healthcare* section below for more details.

Emergency rooms are one of the first steps of the "revolving door" phenomenon, where individuals with severe behavioral health conditions cycle between emergency rooms, hospitals, jails, and homelessness. Thus, each emergency room visit represents a significant opportunity to break that cycle. Given their psychiatric expertise and specialized settings, psychiatric emergency rooms are generally preferred over standard emergency rooms for behavioral health emergencies, if they are available in your community. Psychiatric emergency rooms also tend to have relationships with behavioral health treatment services that may facilitate referrals once someone's psychiatric emergency is stabilized.

Acute Care (Inpatient/Hospital-Based Settings)

Acute psychiatric care involves the treatment of psychiatric needs in inpatient or hospital-based settings. The focus of care in these situations is acute stabilization of severe psychiatric symptoms, dangerousness to oneself or others, and/or the ability to care for oneself. The most typical conditions treated in these settings are psychosis, bipolar disorder, depression, and withdrawal from substances such as alcohol or opioids.

While facility licensure terminology differs between states, acute psychiatric care typically occurs in one of several hospital-based settings, such as hospitals focused on medical conditions (general acute hospitals), those that specialize in psychiatric conditions (acute psychiatric hospitals), or facilities that specialize in substance use disorders (chemical dependency recovery hospitals). Although some acute psychiatric hospitals are located within general acute hospital settings, it is more common for psychiatric hospitals to be freestanding and separate from general acute hospitals.

Additionally, inpatient mental health care is typically delivered in locked settings for individuals on psychiatric holds that are generally up to 72 hours, 14 days, or 30 days or more, depending on one's conservatorship or legal status. Importantly, the duration of psychiatric holds varies by region across the country. Inpatient mental health care can also be provided voluntarily if someone chooses to be treated in that setting (i.e., someone with schizophrenia who has insight and is open to treatment). Unlike inpatient mental healthcare which is most often delivered in locked settings, inpatient substance use care is generally delivered in unlocked settings where clients can voluntarily leave.

Treatment services delivered in inpatient mental health settings typically involve some combination of a multidisciplinary team of psychiatrists, nurse practitioners, physician assistants, nurses, social workers, psychologists, psychiatric technicians, and peer specialists. On the other hand, inpatient substance use settings tend to have less medically trained staff and lower staff ratios compared to inpatient mental health settings, in addition to substance use counselors and physicians with expertise in addiction. The duration of inpatient psychiatric care is typically several days to several weeks, though there are instances where longer-term stays occur given long-term needs and a lack of alternative options in the community.

One of the essential treatment goals in the inpatient setting is to stabilize the acute psychiatric presentation to ready someone for follow-up care in the community. Thus, the medications, individual therapy, group therapy, case management, and recreational activities that characterize treatment in inpatient psychiatric settings are geared toward this aim.

For mental health presentations, stabilization of psychotic, mood, or other symptoms in inpatient settings generally refers to the improvement of immediate symptoms to a point where they can be safely managed outside of the hospital setting, such as in a clinic. For substance use presentations, stabilization often involves controlling symptoms of withdrawal from substances that can make longer-term recovery challenging. While withdrawal from alcohol and sedatives such as benzodiazepines or barbiturates are the main substances that are considered immediately life-threatening, withdrawal from opioids can also be dangerous given the higher likelihood of relapse and overdose when someone is experiencing withdrawal symptoms, particularly given the higher prevalence of high potency opioids such as fentanyl in many communities.

Care in inpatient settings is distinct from other settings. At a high level, a typical day in an inpatient psychiatric setting involves the treating physician or associate rounding on clients in the morning to evaluate for progress, response and side effects to medications, and readiness for discharge to sub-acute or outpatient settings. The outcome is then discussed with other members of the multidisciplinary care team and modified, as needed. The rest of the day is spent implementing the individual treatment plan of clients informed by this daily assessment.

There are several strategies that caregivers can employ to improve care in inpatient mental health and substance use settings. Treatment teams often need to rely on the history they gather from clients themselves, which can sometimes be incomplete or compromised depending on someone's psychiatric presentation. They can also glean a patient's behavioral health history from treatment records collected from prior providers. However, these records are not always immediately available.

As a result, essential information—such as what diagnoses and treatments a client has received in the past, what has been effective and ineffective, and medication side effects— can sometimes be missed.

Caregivers are often in the best position to help organize a client's behavioral health history to support the care team's work. By providing a thorough written history of the client to the treating team to help inform care, as described in Chapter Six, caregivers can provide multiple people on the treatment team with important details to help shape the care of their loved one. They can also capture more nuanced information that oftentimes only caregivers are aware of, while maximizing the likelihood of positive outcomes by helping to inform care decisions by the treatment team.

Although this is not a requirement for good quality care, it can be helpful, particularly if someone has not received their treatment within the same system of care and instead has been treated by multiple providers in different systems.

If staff working in inpatient settings cite HIPAA as a reason why they cannot disclose if someone is a client or share information, see the *Legalities of Behavioral Healthcare* section below for more details on what options you have in these situations.

While medications for addiction treatment, such as buprenorphine and naltrexone, are evidence-based and federally approved for opioid and alcohol use disorders, it is still a commonly under-utilized treatment intervention in substance use settings. When caregivers have loved ones being treated for opioid and/or alcohol use disorders, it is generally prudent to check if medications are available at one's treatment setting for those who are interested in this evidence-based intervention.

While specific substance use settings will indicate that they are a "social model" program (meaning that they primarily rely on counseling or talk therapy) as opposed to a "medical model" program (which offers medications for addiction treatment and/or withdrawal management medications), settings that follow best practices for addiction treatment generally offer "biopsychosocial" programs that provide both therapy and addiction medications. However, many inpatient settings specializing in substance use will have limitations around treating individuals with co-occurring serious mental illness unless their condition is stable, given the types of staff they have working in these settings. Individuals with co-occurring serious mental illness and substance use who require hospital-based care would typically be better served in inpatient mental health settings, as they can often handle the treatment of both conditions better than standalone substance use treatment settings.

The evidence is clear that people with co-occurring mental health and substance use conditions are best served by being treated for their conditions simultaneously as opposed to sequentially. Behavioral health systems are making progress in providing more integrated treatment services for people with co-occurring mental health and substance use conditions. That said, communities that are doing this competently are still more the minority than the majority. For this reason, it is essential to consider what staff and services an inpatient setting offers when determining where someone with co-occurring mental health and substance use conditions would be best served.

Sub-Acute Care (Residential and Non-Hospital-Based Settings)

Sub-acute care typically refers to services provided to individuals who are stable enough to be treated outside of a hospital setting, but not stable enough for lower intensity outpatient (clinic- or community-based) services. Thus, sub-acute psychiatric care is considered a medium level of intensity and occurs in various types of residential settings—some locked and others unlocked. Sub-acute services are also sometimes provided in permanent supportive or transitional housing settings when clinical services are "wrapped around" housing settings. In short, sub-acute services include a combination of a bed to stay in for varied periods of time (typically weeks to months) and treatment services.

Individuals who need more structure and are at risk for leaving treatment against medical advice may be placed in locked residential settings. Others who need sub-acute care but are more stable may be placed in unlocked residential settings. These settings may also include skilled nursing facilities (SNF), particularly for those with co-occurring physical health conditions.

There are various levels of residential treatment and withdrawal management in sub-acute settings focused on substance use disorders. The differences in the various residential substance use disorder treatment settings primarily relate to the types of practitioners available on-site, the intensity and number of hours of services delivered per week, as well as substance use settings that may have particular expertise with treating individuals with co-occurring mental health conditions. Similar to services in other settings, care in sub-acute settings generally involves individual therapy, group therapy, crisis intervention, relapse prevention, medication management, and case management, among other services.

While housing systems are distinct from behavioral health systems in their focus on housing instead of treatment services, there are increasing efforts to better integrate housing and behavioral health systems given the high proportion of people who need both services. Examples of housing settings that are available in many regions across the country and often paired with various forms of health, behavioral health, and social service supports to complement housing needs, include but are not limited to:

- Longer-term housing
- Permanent supportive housing
- Medium-term housing
- Diverse forms of transitional housing
- Board and care settings for people with behavioral health conditions
- Recovery residences for people with substance use disorders

- Single room occupancy (SRO) settings
- Transitional shelters for survivors of domestic violence
- Short-term housing
- Emergency shelters

Individuals with behavioral health conditions residing in these housing options will sometimes have their treatment services layered on top of their housing setting. This layering may mean that clinical services are brought to clients where they reside, or that treatment services are at a clinic with facilitated transportation.

As noted in the other care settings above, caregivers can help enhance outcomes in sub-acute settings by providing a complete history (i.e., a story of their loved one's health status) for the treatment team. This information helps to inform the treatment teams' care decisions, and encourages appropriate care coordination—particularly across different systems such as mental health, substance use, and housing systems.

Outpatient Care (Clinic- or Community-Based Settings)

Outpatient services are typically provided at clinics or in the community as field-based services where providers meet clients wherever they are to deliver their services, instead of providing care in facilities such as hospitals.

While outpatient treatment of mental health and substance use disorders is one of the least intensive levels of care, they are also one of the most important. This is because outpatient treatment is the primary service type for addressing chronic conditions longitudinally. It is also the most readily available setting and is used most frequently given that they don't require the operational expenses associated with 24/7 facilities such as residential or hospital-based care. Individuals served in outpatient settings are generally considered stable and do not need institutional care in hospital or residential settings.

There are different forms of outpatient treatment. Individuals with serious mental illness tend to respond best to a team-based approach with a multidisciplinary team of clinicians and case managers that offer a spectrum of expertise to help support complex clients. These team-based models have evidence to support their efficacy and are typically comprised of a combination of psychiatrists, nurses, psychologists, social workers, marriage and family therapists, and peers with lived experience.

The benefit of this team-based approach is that different care providers on the team often have different strengths and can play different roles to best support the varied needs of clients with serious mental illness. Typical outpatient mental health services occur in either a clinic or field-based setting and involve a treatment team member checking in with the client anywhere from once per month to several times per week or even daily, depending on need. Outpatient services involve a range of services including medication management, individual therapy, group therapy, family therapy, crisis services, coping skills training, care coordination, and case management.

Similar to the variability in outpatient mental health settings, there are also assorted flavors of outpatient substance use treatment. For example, outpatient care can have different intensity levels in substance use systems characterized by higher weekly service hours in intensive outpatient treatment than in standard outpatient substance use treatment, can occur in opioid treatment program settings that offer medications such as methadone and buprenorphine, and can also include outpatient withdrawal management.

The duration of outpatient services is as long as individuals need. For clients with chronic psychiatric conditions that need longitudinal follow-up, outpatient care can be delivered for years or even decades. Given the length of time someone is treated in outpatient settings, the outpatient treatment provider or team is often the person/people caregivers become most familiar with. Ensuring that there is consent to release information to caregivers is vital, assuming the client is agreeable. If not, caregivers can still provide the treatment team with a thorough history of the client's prior care and other pertinent details to inform their care. See the *Legalities of Behavioral Healthcare* section below for more information about relevant history that is often helpful for the clinical team.

Legalities of Behavioral Health Care

Arguably, nowhere else in health care are legalities as intertwined with the delivery of care as in psychiatry and behavioral health, especially for individuals on the more serious end of the behavioral health spectrum. Whether related to confidentiality and information sharing, or psychiatric holds required for instances in which involuntary treatment is clinically appropriate, it is nearly impossible to successfully navigate behavioral health systems without at least a cursory understanding of the laws that govern behavioral healthcare.

An important caveat anytime legalities such as conservatorships and psychiatric holds are discussed in generalities is that various legal regulations and nuances differ by state and local jurisdictions. As a result, details specific to your region will need to be discussed with appropriate professionals familiar with the laws and regulations in your area.

This chapter aims to provide a high-level summary of the most essential legal considerations related to behavioral health that are widely applicable across the United States. Key areas of focus will be confidentiality and addressing instances of involuntary care within the legal framework of both civil and criminal courts.

Confidentiality

As a caregiver, not being able to receive information about a loved one as a result of confidentiality regulations can be one of the most frustrating aspects of the behavioral health journey.

HIPAA is a regulation that governs the use and disclosure of protected health information and ensures that patients understand and are able to control how their health information is used. A key goal of HIPAA is to protect sensitive health information from being disclosed without the patient's consent or knowledge. Another important goal of HIPAA is to establish a mechanism for health information to be appropriately shared to facilitate the provision of coordinated, high-quality health care, and protect the public's health and well-being. HIPAA pertains to all healthcare systems, including the physical and mental health systems, as well as substance use systems.

While HIPAA requires that protected health information is shared with patient consent, there are various exceptions when patient consent is not required to share HIPAA-protected information. These exceptions include disclosing HIPAA protected health information for treatment and coordination purposes (so that treatment providers can share information to inform and coordinate care), administrative purposes (to ensure that payers of health care, such as insurance companies, have the information they need in order to operate), for public health reasons such as mandated reporting of tuberculosis exposures, for research, to make reports to the police, and for medical emergencies.

While there are different situations where HIPAA-protected health information can be shared even without patient consent, adult patients can restrict their providers from releasing their protected health information in most other instances. However, HIPAA does not restrict the health provider from *receiving* information. For example, while a psychiatric hospital would not be able to share adult patient information with caregivers without patient consent, there is nothing preventing caregivers from providing essential information to the psychiatric hospital to inform their loved one's care. This is a common misconception even among mental health providers.

A less well-known confidentiality regulation is the federal rule that guides the use and disclosure of substance use-related information. Known as 42 Code of Federal Regulations (CFR) Part 2, the requirements around sharing and using substance use-related information only pertain to entities that hold themselves out as principally providing substance use treatment. Importantly, a federally qualified health center that does not frame substance use treatment as a principal service, but rather a complementary service to their main focus on primary care, would not need to abide by 42 CFR Part 2, whereas a substance use treatment facility would.

The key difference between HIPAA and 42 CFR Part 2 is that the regulations governing the use and disclosure of substance use information under 42 CFR Part 2 are stricter than HIPAA. While HIPAA allows for the disclosure of information between treatment providers and for care coordination purposes, 42 CFR Part 2 currently does not allow this. Moreover, it prevents this disclosure unless the patient has consented to share their substance use treatment information for these purposes.

Except for a more limited set of exempted circumstances (e.g., medical emergencies, valid court orders requiring the disclosure of substance use information, mandated reporting for child abuse, etc.), 42 CFR Part 2 typically requires patient consent to share substance use treatment information. There are efforts underway at a federal level to better align 42 CFR Part 2 and HIPAA to facilitate more coordinated and integrated behavioral health information exchange, but this is still a work in progress. In either case, similar to HIPAA, 42 CFR Part 2 does not prevent the receipt of substance use related information from caregivers, but rather only the disclosure of substance use information related to the patient without their consent.

States can elect to have more restrictive requirements than what HIPAA and 42 CFR Part require but cannot establish more lenient confidentiality requirements. Various states, such as California, do have stricter requirements than what federal HIPAA regulations allow, but in general, states do not have rules that are stricter than the federal 42 CFR Part 2 requirement, partly because of how strict those Part 2 requirements are already.

Involuntary Care in Behavioral Health

Good behavioral health care aims to empower clients and support the self-determination of their overall health, whether related to mental health, substance use, physical health, housing, or other social determinants of health. This is achieved by having clear and open discussions with clients and, ideally, their caregivers about their care (assuming necessary client consent to release information is obtained), and taking a collaborative decision-making approach that appropriately balances deference to client autonomy, with the recognition that behavioral health practitioners also have a responsibility to use their expertise to improve the health and well-being of their clients. As is the case with quality cancer care, good behavioral health care is multidimensional and is neither the client dictating to their practitioner what treatment they need to provide, nor a practitioner dictating to their client what treatment they need to receive.

While this harmonious picture of healthcare delivery is always ideal and often possible, complexities are introduced when health conditions involving the brain impact the capacity to make reasonable medical decisions. Medical systems have adapted to recognize that brain conditions such as Alzheimer's dementia often rob individuals of the ability to make reasonable medical decisions. There are both accepted practices and formal legal channels to delegate decision-making to families or practitioners, when necessary, to ensure appropriate care is delivered in these instances, even if this care is protested by the individual with Alzheimer's. Although few people would allow their grandmother with dementia to decline care for a treatable condition when she falls in the shower and breaks her arm, if their brother with schizophrenia does the same, physical and mental health systems often cite patient autonomy as reasons to question whether psychiatric care should proceed against their wishes.

There is a thin line between empowering the person and empowering their condition. Since a person is not their condition, these concepts are very different, and allowing individuals with serious mental illness who cannot make reasonable medical decisions to decline psychiatric care often amounts to the empowerment of their condition instead of their person. For this reason, there are various avenues to mandate care for individuals for whom this is necessary and appropriate. Some of these mechanisms reside within civil legal channels, and others follow criminal legal channels.

Importantly, involuntary care is less commonly applied to individuals who primarily have substance use disorders with no co-occurring serious mental illness. There are distinct reasons for this and fundamental differences between the treatment of serious mental illnesses and the treatment of substance use disorders. One of these differences is that substance use disorders are at least twice as common as serious mental illness, and according to federal data, over 95 percent of people with substance use disorders either don't think they need treatment or don't want it.

If people with substance use disorders were routinely compelled into treatment, this would result in an extraordinary increase in involuntary care. Considering that substance use systems have traditionally been underfunded, there would undoubtedly be significant capacity constraints should most people with substance use disorders be mandated to receive care. These constraints would also lead to questions related to equity and which populations are able to access services and more likely to receive involuntary care.

Additionally, recovery from substance use typically requires longer periods of treatment to achieve long-term recovery. While there are federally approved medications for alcohol and opioid use disorders, the effect of those medications on symptoms of substance use disorders (such as cravings) are different than antipsychotics. With antipsychotics, someone can have no intrinsic motivation for treatment but still have psychotic symptoms that improve with antipsychotic medications.

Since there are federally approved medications for only two specific types of addiction, the primary treatment for most people with substance use disorders would be counseling and talk therapy. While effective, counseling and talk therapy require a high level of intrinsic motivation since those that are only superficially engaged are less likely to experience benefits from these interventions. Further, given the unlikely scenario that millions of people with substance use would be involuntarily committed to treatment for extended periods of time, there are reasonable questions about the effectiveness of this approach if involuntary care were routinely applied to people who primarily have substance use disorders with no co-occurring serious mental illness.

Involuntary Psychiatric Care in the Civil Legal System

Within the civil legal system, psychiatric holds, court mandates, and conservatorships are the main options to compel psychiatric care when voluntary options are not viable.

Most states have short-term psychiatric holds that allow for the involuntary evaluation and treatment of individuals who meet the hold criteria, which generally center around imminent dangerousness (danger to self or others) and/or grave disability, which is often defined as the inability to care for oneself because of a mental disorder, as demonstrated by the failure to provide for one's food, shelter, or clothing.

There is often a degree of subjectivity to grave disability criteria, as psychiatrists and assessors frequently have different thresholds for determining when someone cannot care for themselves. For example, one assessor may decide that someone who has schizophrenia and is homeless, eats food out of a trashcan, wears clothes from the streets, and sleeps under a highway overpass, has not met the grave disability criteria. On the other hand, another assessor may conclude that this self-care plan is evidence of the individual's inability to care for themselves.

Similarly, there is also subjectivity related to how imminently dangerous someone may be, with some assessors only triggering dangerousness criteria for psychiatric holds if someone is actively suicidal or homicidal. Other assessors may determine that one meets the dangerousness criteria for a psychiatric hold if they have had recent thoughts or actions that reflect harm to themselves or others.

Given the subjectivity of these determinations, this is an opportunity for caregivers to inform the assessors' perspectives, who often need to rely on the client's word and do not always benefit from information from collateral sources such as caregivers to inform their perspectives.

For example, someone may present completely normal and answer "no" to all dangerousness or grave disability questions. But upon speaking with their family, an assessor may find out that the client hasn't eaten for four days because he believes his family is poisoning his food and has mentioned thoughts of killing himself. This essential information could mean the difference between the assessor determining that a psychiatric hold is inappropriate, versus arriving at the opposite conclusion.

In many states, the duration of these short-term psychiatric holds is up to 72 hours, with the option to present to a judge or hearing officer to pursue temporary extensions for 14 days or more. These temporary psychiatric holds are typically used in acute and crisis situations to more immediately evaluate and treat individuals who would otherwise be unable to care for themselves, or present as a danger to themselves or others.

As a step-up from temporary psychiatric holds, individuals with serious mental illness who require more longitudinal services, but who have not demonstrated a capacity to engage in these services voluntarily, are at times considered for court-ordered outpatient services. These programs are sometimes called outpatient commitment or assisted outpatient treatment (AOT) programs.

The eligibility criteria for AOT programs generally focus on demonstrated recidivism with voluntary psychiatric care characterized by some combination of hospitalizations, emergency room visits, and episodes of incarceration, dangerousness, or grave disability. Specific eligibility criteria vary by region, so one should contact their local mental health system to determine what similar programs are available in their area.

While these programs often involve a spectrum of wraparound services such as medication management, therapy, crisis stabilization, case management, mobile support services, and housing support, there is variability in the services included in these AOT programs. Further, the court order for AOT programs generally either compels treatment or compels an evaluation for a psychiatric hold if an individual were decompensating. In all cases, the goal of these time limited AOT programs is meaningful client engagement. In many instances, the outcome of these programs is voluntary engagement with the care team. Studies of such programs across the U.S. support their effectiveness for a specific subset of individuals with serious mental illness due to what is sometimes called the "black robe effect," where people are sometimes more influenced by what a judge will tell them as opposed to a doctor's recommendations. Research has also demonstrated that AOT programs have been associated with reduced hospitalizations, reduced episodes of incarceration, and enhanced treatment engagement with psychiatric care.

As opposed to voluntary psychiatric services, the other end of the patient autonomy spectrum is legal conservatorships. There are different conservatorship types. One type focuses on financial decisions, while another focuses on medical conditions, called probate conservatorships, including dementia care.

Mental health conservatorships, on the other hand, are court orders that delegate psychiatric care decisions to a conservator who sometimes is a caregiver and a court-appointed public conservator or guardian when the client is a youth. While conserved clients are often served in locked psychiatric settings, consistent with the increasing use of outpatient AOT programs noted above, care for conserved clients is increasingly being provided in outpatient settings to serve people in the least restrictive environment possible. While the duration of a temporary conservatorship is typically a month, longer-term conservatorships can persist for up to a year. When longer-term court orders are needed, conservatorships can be renewed or extended.

Lastly, mental health advance directives are legal documents that describe what one would want to happen should their psychiatric state deteriorate to the point of needing to rely on others to make reasonable psychiatric decisions. This is an under-utilized and essential consideration for many people with behavioral health conditions, and will be covered more in Chapter Seven.

Involuntary Psychiatric Care in the Criminal Legal System

Criminal courts also have different options to encourage psychiatric treatment when individuals with serious mental illness and substance use disorders decline care voluntarily. The most common are diversion programs, such as mental health or drug courts, that offer someone the ability to avoid jail time if they agree to participate in mental health or substance use treatment.

Technically, mental health and drug courts are considered voluntary, given that participants have a choice whether to pursue treatment or to serve their jail time. Still, extrinsic factors motivate participation in these programs, so they're included for consideration in this section.

Evidence supports the effectiveness of mental health and drug courts. While they are not available in every jurisdiction, they are becoming increasingly common in communities across the country.

There are various legal tools to compel treatment when one is criminally charged, incarcerated, or in a state forensic hospital that often serves as a long-term locked treatment for incarcerated individuals with serious mental illness. In most cases, these tools involve court mandates that one must receive treatment even if it is against their wishes. This is used to establish the legal definition of competency to stand trial.

For example, someone who committed armed robbery may have been determined to be incompetent to stand trial and required by court order to receive treatment in a state forensic hospital to restore them to competency to stand trial. Often, if their psychiatric status improves, they will stand trial versus staying in the state forensic hospital on a long-term basis. Given unique legal aspects of each case and regional differences in the approach to these justice-involved court actions, it is recommended that you inquire with legal experts in your area to learn more about these legal considerations.

Behavioral Health Treatment Practitioners

For caregivers looking for behavioral health services for their loved ones, the different types of behavioral health practitioners, their various credentials, and imprecise terminology used in the field, add to the complexity of navigating behavioral health systems. This portion of the chapter provides a foundational understanding of the most common alphabet soup of practitioners in the behavioral health field, while also recognizing that there are regional and state-level differences in some terminology and practitioner credentials.

Practitioner-Related Terminology

While the term *behavioral health* is technically inclusive of both *mental health* and *substance use disorders*, this terminology is sometimes more loosely applied to practitioners even if they do not specialize in clients with both *mental health* and *substance use* conditions, known as *co-occurring* or *dual diagnosis* populations. While co-occurring populations could refer to any combination of conditions (e.g., physical health, mental health, substance use), it often refers to individuals with both mental health and substance use conditions within a behavioral health context. For this reason, if the services and clinical expertise one needs is the treatment of both mental health and substance use conditions, it can be helpful to verify if the behavioral health practitioner you are considering specializes in both and serves co-occurring populations.

Similarly, the term *therapist* or *psychotherapist* is a broad term that describes someone who provides talk therapy. A therapist's background can vary widely, given that different practitioner types such as social workers, marriage and family therapists, psychologists, counselors, and psychiatrists can all provide talk therapy. Suppose one is looking for a therapist of a particular discipline; for example, a therapist that is a psychologist. In that case, the easiest way to determine this is to refer to the acronyms in their title, as noted below in the *Practitioner Types* section below.

The terms *board certified* and *board eligible* refers to certain practitioner types, such as physicians or nurse practitioners. Board-eligible practitioners have completed the prerequisite training to be eligible to take a board certification exam. In contrast, board-certified practitioners have both completed the prerequisite training and passed the board certification exam. The purpose of board certification is to ensure a standard baseline level of knowledge and expertise about the field in which the board exam is focused (e.g., general psychiatry, addiction medicine, etc.). Some good practitioners choose not to take their board certification exam. However, having passed a board certification exam does offer some degree of confidence in one's subject matter expertise.

Finally, while the term *primary care provider* (PCP) or *primary care physician* is generally specific to medical care, it relates to behavioral healthcare, given that there is variability in the extent to which PCPs offer psychiatric and substance use care. A PCP refers to a general practice physician or provider—including nurse practitioners and physician assistants—who provides health care that addresses most patients' needs, instead of specializing in a particular field or area of the body. For example, for common colds, injuries, and other ailments, PCPs typically diagnose and treat the condition, unless the complexity of the situation requires a specialist such as a cardiologist for heart conditions, nephrologist for kidney conditions, etc.

Some PCPs are comfortable and/or trained in addressing behavioral health conditions, including psychiatric and substance use conditions. In these situations, PCPs may deliver these services because they received specialized fellowship training or have a particular interest in that aspect of medicine.

Specialists do not necessarily deliver better care, depending on the condition. One of the many values of PCPs is that they tend to have an integrated view of one's health. This is as opposed to only focusing on one organ or body part. PCPs also tend to develop long-term relationships with their patients, facilitating stronger therapeutic alliances between the care provider and patient. This can improve engagement and communication, which can positively impact health outcomes.

Additionally, PCPs practicing in specific settings, such as *federally qualified health centers* (FQHC), tend to have more familiarity with treating behavioral health conditions due to the patient populations served in those settings. While PCPs tend to focus on individuals with behavioral health conditions on the milder end of the spectrum, their interests and capabilities often vary, and some do care for individuals with serious mental illness or substance use.

PCPs can serve a vital role in caring for someone with behavioral health conditions because sometimes they are the only practitioner a patient trusts or within a geographic area. Other times, the PCP may diagnose someone with a behavioral health condition and then refer them to a psychiatrist or other behavioral health specialist. The PCP may also continue patients on medications once an effective medication regimen is established by a specialist. PCPs are especially important when individuals with behavioral health conditions also have complex medical conditions.

Because of where PCPs are positioned within health systems, they often have an integrated view of one's health and can help manage and coordinate the combination of physical and behavioral health conditions that a patient may have.

Practitioner Types

Below is a list of the most common types of practitioners that deliver behavioral health services, along with their most common credentials to decode the alphabet soup that follows their names:

- **Physicians, including psychiatrists:** Doctor of Medicine (MD), Doctor of Osteopathy (DO)
- **Nurse Practitioners:** Family Nurse Practitioner (FNP), Psychiatric Mental Health Nurse Practitioner (PMHNP), Board Certified Psychiatric Mental Health Nurse Practitioner (PMHNP-BC)
- **Physician Assistants:** Certified Physician Assistants (PA-C), Registered Physician Assistant-Certified (RPA-C)
- **Psychologists:** Doctor of Psychology (PsyD), Doctor of Philosophy in Psychology (PhD)
- **Social Workers:** Bachelor of Social Work (BSW), Associate of Social Work (ASW), Master of Social Work (MSW), Doctor of Philosophy in Social Work (Ph.D.), Doctor of Social Work (DSW)
- **Marriage and Family Therapists:** Associate Marriage and Family Therapist (AMFT), Marriage and Family Therapist (MFT), Doctor of Philosophy in Marriage and Family Therapy (PhD), Doctor of Marriage and Family Therapy (DMFT)
- **Substance Use Counselors:** Registered Alcohol and Drug Trainee (RADT), Certified Alcohol and Drug Counselor (CADC), Licensed Clinical Alcohol and Drug Counselor (LCADC)
- **Counselors:** Licensed Professional Counselor (LPC), Licensed Professional Clinical Counselor (LPCC), Licensed Clinical Professional Counselor (LCPC), Licensed Mental Health Counselor (LMHC), and Licensed Clinical Mental Health Counselor (LCMHC)

NOTE: Different states use different credentials to demonstrate their training. While this list includes examples of various counselor credentials from most regions across the United States, it is not exhaustive.

A key point of confusion regarding practitioners is how they differ in their expertise and service offerings. One of the more common misunderstandings involves the difference between psychiatrists and psychologists, with the primary difference being the type of training they receive.

Psychiatrists graduate from medical school and receive residency training in psychiatric medicine to prevent, diagnose, and treat behavioral health disorders. They have expertise in prescribing psychiatric medications and receive training in talk therapy. Psychologists specialize in the science of behaviors, emotions, and thoughts, and are also trained in talk therapy. Psychologists can also prescribe medications with specialized experience and training in certain states. In general, psychiatrists will have more experience and training in prescribing psychiatric medications, while psychologists will have more experience and training with talk therapy.

When it comes to nursing practitioners and physician assistants, both can prescribe medications and generally need to practice under the supervision of a physician. The primary difference between psychiatrists and their nurse practitioner and physician assistant colleagues is in training. Nurse practitioners and physician assistants do not complete medical school and receive other types of advanced training.

Payers and Insurance

Understanding the basics of how health systems are financed can be helpful when navigating care for someone with a behavioral health condition. Health systems are typically comprised of providers that deliver the service, and payers that pay the providers to deliver the service. Occasionally, the same entity that is the healthcare provider is also the payer.

Payers are generally governmental entities and/or managed care organizations (commonly also called health insurance companies or health plans) that receive public and/or private/commercial funding to reimburse providers for services provided to members of the managed care organization. Governmental payers include programs such as Medicaid (for low-income individuals), Medicare (for individuals with a disability over age 65), and Veteran's Affairs (for current and former members of the military). Private health insurance companies are the payers with the greatest name recognition given that they commonly advertise their services via commercials and are the entities that the public generally interacts with when managing their bills for health services. The last payer type is less common and known as self-pay for individuals with the means to pay for their health care directly without relying on insurance.

There are different ways to pay for health care services, including cost-based models that pay providers based on the cost of delivering those services, fee-for-service models that pay for each service, and managed care models that attempt to balance the costs, quantity, and quality of services via utilization controls and various complex reimbursement approaches. Given that most health systems in the United States operate via managed care principles, including behavioral health systems, this will be the focus of this chapter.

There are various types of managed care plan models:

Health Maintenance Organization (HMO): HMO plans typically have the lowest out-of-pocket expenses because the plan negotiates discounted fees with specific networks of providers to deliver services to its members. However, these lower fees are only available to members when they are served by providers that are in-network (providers that are approved to deliver services in their network), and services outside of this network (out-of-network) are often not covered. HMO plans also generally require a primary care provider to refer someone to a specialist if they need specialty services. Overall, HMOs typically offer the lowest costs but are also the least flexible.

Preferred Provider Organization (PPO): Similar to HMOs, PPO plans also establish negotiated rates with in-network providers that can offer lower prices for members. However,

PPO plans offer more flexibility than HMOs by allowing members to receive services from out-of-network providers with the understanding that they will pay more out-of-pocket for this flexibility. PPOs also do not usually require a primary care referral for specialty services. Typically, PPOs tend to cost the most, but also offer more flexibility for members to choose their desired provider.

Exclusive Provider Organization (EPO): EPO plans also establish in-network providers that can offer lower out-of-pocket expenses for their members, but often do not cover any costs of out-of-network providers. EPOs also generally do not require a primary care referral for specialty services. In general, EPO plans are more costly than HMOs but less costly than PPOs and offer flexibility in terms of enabling access to specialists without a primary care referral but no flexibility in terms of paying for out-of-network providers.

Point of Service (POS): POS plans also offer lower prices for in-network providers but allow out-of-network care with higher out-of-pocket expenses. Primary care referrals to specialists are required for POS plans. Overall, out-of-pocket expenses for POS plans are typically higher than HMOs and EPOs, but lower than PPOs. POS plans also offer comparable flexibility as PPOs in terms of out-of-network providers, but less flexibility compared to PPOs with respect to still requiring primary care referrals for specialty services.

There is significant variability in benefits, out-of-pocket expenses, and coverage for out-of-network providers between managed care plan types. As such, the ideal plan is dependent on individual preferences and circumstances. It is advisable to explore available in-network providers in your area for whichever managed care plan type you are considering selecting to ensure comfort with your in-network options. In general, HMOs are the lowest cost, PPOs and POS plans are the most flexible in terms of out-of-network providers, and PPOs and EPOs are the most flexible in terms of not requiring referrals from primary care to see a specialist.

At its core, managed care is a way to manage the balance between controlling healthcare costs while also ensuring quality services. This is often accomplished by establishing utilization controls over reimbursed services, including requirements around eligibility and determining what services are clinically needed, which is often equated with medical necessity.

In managed care systems, an entity such as the government or an employer pays managed care organizations to be responsible for making healthcare services available to their constituents. In turn, managed care organizations contract with a network of providers to deliver these healthcare services and require that members receive services from these network providers to have their health care paid for, either in whole or in part. Services delivered by out-of-network providers will typically either not be covered or will come with more out-of-pocket expenses. Managed care organizations also establish utilization management controls to review care requests to ensure they are medically necessary before they will agree to reimburse providers for services.

While medical necessity at the provider level is a clinical determination of need, medical necessity at the level of the managed care organization is often a blend of clinical need combined with financial considerations related to what will be reimbursed. While these perspectives of medical necessity would ideally be consistent, this is not always the case. Managed care models have at times been criticized for prioritizing their finances over care and denying reimbursement for services that clinicians think should be covered.

This is particularly problematic in the behavioral health field given the high cost of individuals with serious mental illness, and the fact that managed care organizations are often pay for services via a capitated rate, meaning that they are paid the same amount for an individual member whether they require one service or ten services. While this capitated payment model incentivizes value and financial efficiency and may work well for healthier populations, for populations that need a lot of healthcare services, capitated models can also incentivize cost-cutting at the expense of care if appropriate checks and balances are not instituted.

Gary Tsai, M.D.

With this aim in mind, the Mental Health Parity Act, in 1996, and the Mental Health Parity Act and Addiction Equity Act (MHPAEA), in 2008, were federal laws intended to ensure that insurance companies offer similar covered benefits for mental health and substance use conditions as other medical conditions. The goal of the MHPAEA was to prevent scenarios in which insurance companies discriminated against their members with behavioral health conditions by limiting the scope of behavioral health conditions they would cover, or by covering a benefit but establishing utilization controls that were more restrictive than equivalent physical health needs.

While the MHPAEA has been in place for over a decade, it has become clear that enforcement of the requirements of the MHPAEA by insurance companies has been inadequate. Some reasons for this are because insurance companies will sometimes offer a service as a covered benefit but restrict that service through their authorization process, or violate parity requirements by covering only a portion of a behavioral health service even though they cover the complete service needed for an equivalent physical health condition.

Unfortunately, when one speaks with family members of individuals with serious mental illness and other behavioral health conditions, it becomes clear that insurance companies declining to pay for a behavioral health condition is a common occurrence and a substantive barrier to care. When care is denied by an insurance company's determination as opposed to the judgment of a treating clinician, there are opportunities to appeal these denials with the insurance company. In these instances, it can be helpful for caregivers to provide the treatment team with a comprehensive history and understanding of the client's prior psychiatric history and current reason for presentation to care. Refer to Chapter Six on *How to be an Effective Advocate* for more details.

Chapter Five

Getting Help and Treatment Options

Finding a Good Clinician and Clinical Team

Perhaps one of the most important considerations related to behavioral health outcomes is the quality of one's primary behavioral health provider and their clinical team. Whenever possible, it is ideal to speak with or meet your loved one's treatment provider to determine fit with respect to what you and your loved one are looking for in a clinician.

Like other service-oriented professions, asking trusted healthcare providers or friends for recommendations for behavioral health practitioners they would entrust the care of their loved ones to can be another valuable perspective to consider.

Nowadays, many practitioners have their own professional websites or some other footprint on the Internet that provides a sense of who they are, what services they offer, their approach to care, and any populations or areas of practice they specialize in. While online forums with reviews can be helpful, it's also important to note that many times, the reviews that are provided represent the extremes of one's experience, as many people only post reviews when they have a very positive or very negative experience. Additionally, these types of reviews often only describe one side of a given situation and thus may be subjectively or objectively inaccurate.

Identifying a great clinician is not an exact science. However, certain attributes are generally universally appreciated and might suggest a strong clinician.

One foundational asset of a good clinician is being a strong communicator. We've all spoken to healthcare providers that made us feel like they didn't have time for us, and others that made us feel like we were the only patient on their schedule that day. We have also probably interacted with people who sounded intelligent but didn't communicate in a manner that we understood. Clinicians that are strong communicators typically demonstrate that they are willing to spend time explaining things in a clear, thoughtful, comprehensive, and understandable manner. You should understand what your clinician is saying. If you don't and ask for clarification, strong communicators will be able to translate complex behavioral health considerations into more simple and understandable terms.

Another sign of a strong clinician is someone who approaches health care from a collaborative rather than a siloed perspective. While some clinicians prefer to work in isolation, in increasingly complex and integrated healthcare systems that consider someone's whole-person health (physical health, mental health, substance use) and also social determinants of health such as housing/employment/education access/etc., clinicians that value the work and opinions of others in the health and social service professions will be in a better position to deliver high-quality care and coordinate with others in necessary ways. These clinicians also tend to have more holistic views of behavioral health and well-being, recognizing that titrating medication doses is only one component of comprehensive and effective care. One can get a sense of how holistic a clinician's perspective is by asking them about their approach to care and what they do to help their clients when they have health or social issues beyond what they typically focus on. It is ideal for clinicians to be involved with coordinating care with other types of providers, as opposed to simply providing a resource list for clients or families to follow up on their own.

While experience is essential, and good clinicians often have an expansive spectrum of experiences, it's also important to hire a clinician who does not rely solely on their prior experiences and is interested in evolving their knowledge as the field evolves. While new clinicians can sometimes not have sufficient expertise to inform the care of complex clients, clinicians later in their careers can also have difficulty staying abreast of the latest updates in the field. Finding a clinician that is balanced in their experience while maintaining a learner's mindset is often the sign of a quality practitioner.

Similar to the strategy for effective job interviews, identifying the areas or attributes of potential concern for a prospective clinician and then asking questions about them (e.g., asking someone early in their career what experiences they've had treating clients with the unique issues of your loved one, or asking someone how they stay on top of new developments in the psychiatric field) can yield important insights into the fit and quality of a given behavioral health practitioner you are considering working with.

Some situations and cases require clinicians with uncommon expertise. Suppose your loved one needs specialized expertise given the unique circumstances of their case, such as having a rare condition that is contributing to their psychiatric symptoms. In this example, unique subject matter expertise can be another important determining factor in your selection of a clinician.

While board certification for applicable practitioner types is not a prerequisite to being a good clinician, it can suggest at least a baseline level of expertise and is another factor to consider.

Lastly, while peer specialists are distinct from treatment practitioners, they can play an important role in one's recovery and exert significant influence on clients. It is hard to know what it is like to be treated for a behavioral health condition without experiencing it yourself, and peer specialists can be a major strength for care teams and clients alike. Peer specialists can play critical roles by establishing trust and essential therapeutic bonds with clients based on their shared lived experience and helping to educate practitioners about the experience as well. Instances when peer specialists are less helpful are when their perspective is entirely influenced by their own recovery journey, instead of using their experiences to inform a client's journey and recognizing that each recovery journey is different. For example, at times, peer specialists who have achieved recovery without using medications may counsel clients that recovery is possible without using medications given that they recovered without medications, and either intentionally or unintentionally influence the client's decision about taking psychiatric medications. While inappropriate medications are harmful, so is stopping beneficial medications. As such, while peer specialists are without a doubt a value-add to care teams, it is sensible for caregivers to understand both the significant benefits and potential drawbacks of peer specialists, and work with them and their care team if issues arise that may influence client care in suboptimal ways.

Diagnostic Options

When someone you care about begins exhibiting signs and symptoms of what seems like a psychiatric disorder, obtaining an accurate diagnosis is an important first step in determining the most appropriate treatment and next steps. The Diagnostic and Statistical Manual of Mental Disorders (DSM) is commonly known as the "bible" of psychiatric conditions and includes the criteria used to diagnose mental health and substance use disorders. While the DSM can be a helpful tool for caregivers to learn about what factors are considered in specific psychiatric conditions, since its criteria are simultaneously straightforward and complicated with jargon and other nuanced clinical considerations, it is important for qualified practitioners to make diagnoses.

In general, the diagnostic process involves taking a detailed history of someone's life up until the assessment, including their childhood, medical conditions, family history, current signs and symptoms, and other psychosocial considerations that contribute to one's behavioral health. While interviewing and assessing the client themselves is helpful, if someone's mental state is such that an accurate history cannot be obtained, collateral information from caregivers or others from the client's support network becomes essential. Family history and substance use history can be particularly enlightening and not always available to evaluators when they interview the client directly. The diagnostic process may also include laboratory studies to rule out nutritional deficiencies or medical conditions that may contribute to psychiatric presentations, such as thyroid and kidney irregularities.

Although brain imaging such as computed tomography (CT) or magnetic resonance imaging (MRI) is sometimes used to exclude organic causes of psychiatric symptoms, it is not typically used as a first-line diagnostic tool. This is because while studies have demonstrated associations between certain structural brain features and psychiatric illness, the associations have largely not proven to be causal, meaning that psychiatric conditions have not been proven to lead to changes in brain features or vice versa.

For example, studies of individuals with schizophrenia have found reductions in certain brain areas such as cortical gray matter, the hippocampus, amygdala, and frontal and temporal lobes, along with increases in space in the brain such as the ventricles. However, none of these findings are diagnostic, as some of these findings can be accounted for by normal variations in brains from individuals without psychiatric conditions, or can be associated with other conditions such as dementia. There are also certain drawbacks to brain imaging that need to be considered, such as radiation from CT scans, cost, or finding benign anomalies that result in further medical workups that may have adverse outcomes or side effects.

Consequently, while brain imaging is rapidly advancing and may one day become a primary means of diagnosing psychiatric conditions, there are presently limitations in technology and in the science and knowledge of the brain that prevent it from being a primary tool in mainstream psychiatric diagnoses. Until brain imaging allows clinicians to translate findings into actionable clinical decisions, it will largely be limited in its diagnostic use to situations when unusual aspects of a presentation warrant investigation beyond the typical psychiatric diagnostic workup. As such, psychiatric diagnoses are presently primarily clinical diagnoses based on a detailed history, physical, and analysis of presenting signs and symptoms.

In instances where a diagnosis is questioned, before obtaining a second opinion, one may consider inquiring with the original assessor to determine the considerations that contributed to their initial diagnosis. Given the criticality of client history and the details of their signs and symptoms that may not always be available to the evaluator, ensuring that collateral information from caregivers is considered can be essential in facilitating an accurate diagnosis. For this reason, verifying that the original assessor had access to essential information during the diagnostic process is the first step to an accurate diagnosis. If this is not an option, obtaining a second opinion from a different behavioral health practitioner, with access to the important context from the client, pertinent medical and psychiatric records, and collateral information from caregivers and social networks, can help inform the diagnostic picture and subsequent treatment plan.

Treatment Options

At the most fundamental level, good psychiatric care requires two things:

- A good behavioral health practitioner and/or team; and
- Clinically appropriate care delivered in a manner that

facilitates trust and a strong therapeutic alliance or relationship between the treatment practitioner/team and client.

The beginning of Chapter Five, which covers *Finding a Good Clinician and Clinical Team,* highlights some of the most critical elements in identifying a good behavioral health practitioner and/or team. Importantly, finding a behavioral health practitioner and/or team is as much about the client as it is about the practitioner/team. For example, certain people gravitate and connect better with certain attributes or demographics that may influence the therapeutic alliance between a treatment provider or team and the client, so these are important variables to consider.

For the second element of good psychiatric care noted above, clinically appropriate care looks different for everyone. Some instances involve participation in a particular program or receiving a particular medication or formulation of medication (long-acting injection versus oral pills).

While outlining all potential clinical considerations in the care of someone with serious mental illness is outside the scope of this book, some of the most critical concerns in determining what treatment might work best for a given individual are noted below.

Firstly, studies have consistently demonstrated that talk therapy, in combination with clinically appropriate psychiatric medications, increases the likelihood of long-term recovery for individuals with serious mental illness as compared to either intervention alone. While some individuals may not want or be in a psychiatric state to meaningfully participate in talk therapy, it can be an incredibly powerful therapeutic tool for the right client. There are different approaches to talk therapy, also commonly referred to as psychotherapy, which is generally based on one of five theories:

Psychoanalytic and psychodynamic therapy – This approach to therapy relies on changing problematic thoughts, feelings, or behaviors by uncovering meanings and motivations that are often sub-conscious and not readily apparent to people. One of the vehicles by which these sub-conscious issues are explored is through the relationship and interactions between the therapist and client.

Behavioral therapy – This therapy technique focuses on learned behaviors and training oneself to learn desired behaviors and unlearn counterproductive ones through various types of conditioning, including the use of rewards and punishments.

Cognitive therapy – This approach to therapy is grounded in the belief that dysfunctional thinking leads to undesired feelings and behaviors. Changing this dysfunctional thinking is the key to establishing greater control over one's undesirable feelings and actions.

Importantly, cognitive behavioral therapy (CBT) is a common form of talk therapy that combines cognitive and behavioral therapeutic techniques, focusing on both thoughts and behaviors to influence one's feelings.

Humanistic therapy – Empowering clients through support and concern is the general focus of this therapeutic approach. Self-determination and emphasizing the capacity for clients to make rational decisions to optimize their potential is also a hallmark of this approach to therapy.

Integrative therapy – Similar to how no one is identical, practitioners of integrative therapy braid elements of different therapy techniques together to best meet clients' individualized needs.

Because different people prefer and respond to different psychotherapeutic approaches, there is no particular type of talk therapy that is best. But generally, evidence and experience support the idea that individuals with serious mental illness can do well with talk therapy that is both structured and flexible enough to adapt to evolving needs. For this reason, CBT, humanistic and supportive therapy approaches, and various permutations of these techniques are often ideal for individuals with conditions on the more severe end of the psychiatric spectrum.

When it comes to psychiatric medications, while there is sometimes an aversion to using medications to treat psychiatric conditions that often do not exist with other medical conditions, the reality is that medications are an important and necessary element of treatment for a substantial proportion of people with serious mental illness..

Psychiatric prescribers typically have different approaches to medication management. Some prefer to start at low doses and titrate the dose up slowly. In contrast, others want to maximize medication doses according to what is tolerable for an individual, depending on side effects, to maximize effectiveness quickly. Given how side effects can be the difference between someone taking their medications consistently and not, the more common prescribing approach is to offer the lowest effective dose.

The side effects of psychiatric medications may include potential sedation, weight gain, movement disorders (e.g., tremors, involuntary movements), headache, increased cholesterol or triglycerides in the blood, and dry mouth. Notably, while the lists of potential side effects in medication packaging often identify every possible side effect that has been associated with a particular medication, similar to the required list of possible side effects noted in many ads for medications on TV, in the majority of clinical instances, less than a handful of those side effects occur with most clients. Additionally, starting medications for any condition must consider both the potential side effects of the medication as well as the benefits of the medication, including the risks of not treating someone with medication.

For individuals with serious mental illness, another important medication-related consideration is that there are different formulations of psychiatric medications such as pills, liquids, dissolvable tablets or film, or long-acting injectable formulations that may only require one injection every several weeks or months, depending on the specific medicine. This is essential to consider because different medication formulations may impact adherence to the medication, and adherence often directly impacts the effectiveness of treatment.

A medication that is not taken does not have the opportunity to work. Since pills sometimes need to be taken several times per day and may be forgotten or more easily avoided when individuals with serious mental illness do not believe they need medications, formulations of medications that are easier to administer may help ensure that an individual receives the required medications. For example, long-acting injectable medications that may stay in someone's system for weeks or months removes the daily worry of whether someone took their medications. Generally, before someone is provided a long-acting medication, they are first administered formulations of the same medication orally, to ensure that it is well-tolerated and has no allergic or significant adverse effects.

Unfortunately, identifying the best medication for someone is often trial and error, as science and medicine are not at a state yet where someone's lab results or genetics can reveal what medication they would definitively respond best to. However, each medication has a profile of commonly associated benefits and side effects, and a good prescriber will be familiar with and consider these various benefits and side effects to match clients with trying the medication that will most likely yield benefits with the least amount of side effects. This risk-benefit analysis is essential for any medication, and good prescribers will often describe their rationale for choosing a particular medication.

When comparing the effectiveness of older (first) versus newer (second) generation antipsychotics, there are more similarities than differences. The main exception is the antipsychotic called clozapine, which was the first second-generation psychotic that was developed.

Clozapine has been shown to be the most effective antipsychotic, including in instances when patients have not responded to other antipsychotic medications. It has also been demonstrated to reduce suicidal and violent behaviors in certain individuals. However, the reason why clozapine is generally not the first antipsychotic medication that is tried is given its side effect profile, which includes usual antipsychotic side effects of sedation, weight gain, movement disorders, etc., in addition to a more serious blood condition called agranulocytosis, which results in reduced white blood cells and can make people more prone to potentially life-threatening infections. Because of this risk, clients who are prescribed clozapine must take weekly blood tests for the first six months, then every other week for six months, with the gradual ability to take a blood test monthly thereafter, assuming no emergence of agranulocytosis.

Despite the potentially serious side effects, clozapine and other antipsychotics can also be lifesaving. This is why a thoughtful risk-benefit analysis is essential in each individualized clinical case to inform the prescribing process.

Different antipsychotic medications have different profiles of benefits and risks, and some are more appropriate depending on the patient and symptoms. Depending on the way they work (their mechanisms of action) and the neurotransmitters that the antipsychotic medication targets in specific areas of the brain, there are situations where the risk and benefit profiles for certain antipsychotics better match a given client based on their individualized clinical need. It is helpful to talk through these considerations with your psychiatrist or prescriber.

Psychiatric medications and psychotherapy are by far the most common treatments for individuals with serious mental illness and other psychiatric conditions. As a result, they have a longer track record demonstrating a favorable risk and benefit profile. For these reasons, medications and psychotherapy should be considered first-line treatment options for individuals with serious mental illness and other psychiatric conditions.

As far as procedural interventions for psychiatric disorders, electroconvulsive therapy (ECT) is a procedure that involves brief electrical stimulation of the brain while someone is under anesthesia, and is most commonly used to treat severe depression or bipolar disorder. It is also used for catatonia and treatment-resistant psychosis. The exact mechanism by which ECT works is unknown. However, it is thought to essentially "reset" and normalize activities in key areas of the brain involved with mood and emotional regulation.

The procedure nowadays is much different than "electroshock therapy" in the past, as people are asleep and under anesthesia with modern ECT. The procedure is brief, with clients waking up after only five to ten minutes. Typically, individuals receiving ECT will receive between four to a dozen treatments, with some receiving periodic ECT treatments every month or several months. Although the most concerning side effect of ECT is often memory loss, modern ECT that uses unilateral electrodes over the nondominant half of the brain help to minimize this adverse effect. In general, ECT is more accepted and commonly used in Europe, given negative publicity about the procedure in the United States. ECT can be an important option to consider if antipsychotic medications, including clozapine, do not provide clinical benefit in particular cases.

Transcranial magnetic stimulation (TMS) is a non-invasive procedure that involves placing an electromagnetic coil against the scalp to painlessly deliver a magnetic pulse that stimulates targeted regions of the brain. Unlike with ECT, individuals who receive TMS are awake throughout the procedure, typically lasting between 30 to 60 minutes. TMS has been most studied for the treatment of depression and has demonstrated benefits for this condition. While some studies indicate potential benefit for schizophrenia or OCD, TMS has only minimally been studied for these conditions and is still not readily used for psychiatric conditions beyond depression. TMS is typically well tolerated with minimal side effects.

Other procedures such as vagus nerve stimulation (VNS) and deep brain stimulation (DBS) are less common but have also demonstrated some promise in treating certain psychiatric conditions.

VNS involves implanting an electric pulse generator in the upper chest to stimulate the vagus nerve, which carries messages to brain regions responsible for mood and other functions. Although VNS has only been approved to treat severe depression and medical conditions such as epilepsy, it is being studied for other psychiatric conditions.

DBS is a neurosurgical procedure that involves implanting an electrode to stimulate specific regions of the brain. Given that DBS is a surgical procedure, it is typically reserved for severe cases that have not responded to other available treatment options. This treatment option was first proven for severe movement disorders such as Parkinson's Disease and essential tremors. After success with these conditions, DBS was subsequently studied with a meaningful effect for treatment-resistant depression and obsessive-compulsive disorder (OCD). Some evidence also suggests potential benefits with Tourette's syndrome, Alzheimer's dementia, and addiction.

Treatment Programs

In addition to the clinical considerations of specific treatment options, such as medications, psychotherapy, or non-invasive or invasive procedures that can be tried to better treat individuals with serious mental illness, the program within which these clinical services are delivered is also important to optimize outcomes.

The most common type of program used to support individuals with serious mental illnesses is team-based programs that include various practitioners and care providers from different disciplines. These care teams include peers, case managers, social workers, marriage and family therapists, psychologists, nurse practitioners or physician assistants, and psychiatrists. Although these programs go by different names, Assertive Community Treatment (ACT) or Full-Service Partnerships (FSP) are more well-known terms for this team-based, wraparound approach to care.

The ACT and FSP concept is evidence-based, and these programs are typically mobile and strive to meet clients where they are, both figuratively and literally. Services are varied and flexible and include medication management, talk therapy, crisis intervention, care coordination and case management, housing support, among other services. One of the key objectives of ACT and FSP teams is to help stabilize individuals with serious mental illness in the community so that they do not require institutional or facility-based care, and they generally check in with clients at least once or more per week, titrating the frequency of their encounters based on need.

On any treatment team, someone generally steps in to lead, coordinate, or take a special interest in a particular client. Sometimes this is the team lead, but sometimes it's someone else on the team, such as a care manager or peer specialist. For caregivers, it is often helpful to identify the "champion" for their loved one within any treatment team, and to focus on connecting with both the "champion" and the "team lead" in instances where they may seem to be different individuals within the care team.

Given how common co-occurring mental health conditions are with substance use disorders, programs that specialize in both types of behavioral health care are surprisingly uncommon. One of the reasons for this is because there are often different workforces that treat these conditions—while substance use counselors and addiction specialists primarily treat substance use disorders, the licensed clinicians (e.g., social workers, marriage and family therapists, psychologists) that primarily staff mental health centers don't always have deep familiarity with or an interest in the treatment of substance use disorders.

However, as health systems evolve and the appreciation of the importance of behavioral health care grows, systems, programs, and workforces are increasingly being blended to ensure that programs can effectively treat both mental health and substance use disorders simultaneously. This trend will likely continue as systems and those that work in those systems gear up to provide more whole-person care.

While sometimes called co-occurring or dual diagnosis programs, these programs often have different names. The best way to identify them in your local jurisdiction is to ask if there are programs or members of the care team that specialize in co-occurring populations that have both mental health and substance use disorders. Often, these programs will take an integrated approach that addresses both conditions simultaneously, as evidence supports that this approach is more likely to yield positive outcomes than requiring that someone's substance use be addressed first before their mental health condition is treated, or vice versa.

An increasingly common service that specifically focuses on individuals with psychosis are early psychosis or first-episode psychosis programs (collectively referred to as early psychosis programs here). The underlying premise of these programs is the belief that the trajectory of psychosis can be improved the earlier it is identified and treated. Various studies have demonstrated this, suggesting that early psychosis programs may improve symptoms and functional outcomes, reduce relapses, and prevent or improve disability among people with psychosis when care is begun early during its course.

Early psychosis programs typically aim to engage individuals at their first psychotic break, and combine various evidence-based interventions for psychosis into a program that follows clients two to three years following the onset of their psychotic symptoms. These interventions include low-dose antipsychotics, cognitive and behavioral psychotherapy, family education and support, educational and vocational rehabilitation, and a recovery-oriented, team-based, and collaborative approach to care.

Within early psychosis programs, this team-based approach to early psychosis is sometimes called coordinated specialty care (CSC). It resembles other team-based approaches mentioned above, such as ACT or FSP programs. The key differences between CSC and ACT or FSP programs are related to population, as CSC tends to engage younger individuals with less disability compared to ACT or FSP programs. The duration of services also differs, as CSC programs typically have a two- to three-year commitment after the onset of psychotic symptoms, whereas ACT and FSP programs will often follow individuals for longer periods of time.

While early psychosis programs are not available in every jurisdiction across the U.S., they are becoming more mainstream. When early psychosis programs are not available in your area, one can engage early with your local behavioral health department to seek a multidisciplinary team to provide a similar suite of services as what CSC offers, while simultaneously advocating for the consideration to establish such programs.

Unfortunately, crisis and involuntary services are a common component of care for individuals with more severe behavioral health conditions. There are various important considerations to keep in mind when accessing these services. See the *Crisis Response* and *Involuntary Care in Behavioral Health* section of Chapter Four, respectively, for more information on these topics.

Chapter Six

Effective Advocacy as a Caregiver

There are many ways to be an effective advocate for a loved one with a severe behavioral health condition.

At the clinical level, one can directly influence the care of your loved one through communication with the care team. Another way to be an effective advocate is at a policy level, by influencing the delivery of care for others, including your loved one.

At a clinical level, documenting and communicating both historical and present information with the care team can be one of the most important roles caregivers play in their loved one's care. Caregivers often know those they are caring for better than anyone else. Because members on the care team primarily rely on information gathered from others—whether the client or others—having information from caregivers can be invaluable to inform practitioner care decisions.

Having an accurate clinical history of the story and course of one's behavioral health condition is the single most important foundation to making good care decisions. As a result, keeping a detailed record of your loved one's behavioral health condition can be immensely helpful, both for them to track details themselves and to share with the care team to inform current and future treatment decisions.

While keeping medical records of prior treatment episodes is helpful, even more useful is keeping an organized log of a loved one's behavioral health condition, which can become a living health document that provides all future care practitioners an immediate and accurate picture of their client's behavioral health history. Further, organizing these notes in a way that is easy to understand, and similar to how behavioral health practitioners organize their clinical case formulations, will increase the likelihood that they are incorporated into the individual's official clinical records.

Components of a clinical history that can be included in a write-up for care teams

1. **History of Current Presentation**
   - Describe the present signs and symptoms of concern (e.g., when the signs and symptoms first started, how long they last for, if they respond to anything that makes them better or worse, or any associations or patterns that relate to the individual's presentation)

2. **Past Psychiatric History**
   - Treatment history, if applicable, including names and contacts of prior treatment providers
   - Current and prior psychiatric diagnoses, as applicable
   - Prior suicide attempts, self-harm, or other concerning history
   - History of substance use

3. **Medications**
   - Current and prior medications, including medication names, dosages, and what seemed to work or not work

4. **Medical History**
   - Prior medical conditions, particularly those that may be considered with the prescribing of psychiatric conditions (e.g., heart conditions, diabetes, high blood pressure, high cholesterol, seizures or other neuro-logical conditions, strokes, brain tumors)

5. **Allergies** (both to medications and food)

6. **Family History**
   - Family history of medical, psychiatric, and substance use conditions

7. **Social History**
   - Relevant social history, such as current profession (unemployed/school/work), education level, relevant support system and relationships with family/friends/social networks, activities that provide joy and fulfillment, goals, things that are important to the individual, etc.

8. **Assessment and Plan**
   - What you as a caregiver suspect may be contributing to the signs and symptoms noted above
   - Key interventions that you as a caregiver think may be helpful

Providing this history to new care team members or practitioners can help to communicate important information to ensure that their formulations of the case are informed by your lived experiences with your loved one. While much of the information in this narrative likely will not change, given that they are historical in nature, new details can be added as new information becomes available to keep this history up to date. In this way, this narrative can serve as a living document that contains the most relevant details related to one's care.

Importantly, the more succinct the history, the more likely it will be digested and used by behavioral health practitioners, so it is often beneficial to be as concise as possible.

In addition to this written summary, it is also important for caregivers to build a relationship with the care team, assuming appropriate boundaries. While the therapeutic relationship between client and care team is central, caregivers also play an important role as a rich source of collateral information for the care team to draw from to inform their care decisions. Sometimes, scheduling a regular check-in with the care team, preferably with the client, as appropriate, can ensure regular touch bases between all parties.

As is the case with all health information, abiding by confidentiality regulations is an essential requirement, whether related to HIPAA or the more restrictive regulations governing confidentiality related to substance use conditions known as 42 CFR Part 2. Please refer to the *Confidentiality* section of Chapter Four for more details.

Few people know the challenges, gaps in care, and opportunities to improve services better than individuals with lived experience, such as those with severe behavioral health conditions and their caregivers. As a result, in addition to the individual-level advocacy noted above, caregivers also often play an important role in broader policy changes and reforms at all levels (federal, state, and local) that improve behavioral health services. There are often local behavioral health advocacy circles that one can connect with by contacting your local chapter of the National Alliance on Mental Illness (NAMI), family support groups offered by treatment facilities or behavioral health agencies, or social media groups focused on similar topics. These can be great places to connect with other caregivers who have been through similar experiences for support and advice.

Chapter Seven

Planning Ahead

Against All Odds

Managing a severe behavioral condition can be overwhelming. Once past the immediate challenges of grasping what is going on, inevitable associated emotions, and working through the challenges of accessing care, there are a few other considerations that may help to reduce future stress and complexities.

Advance Directives

Advance directives are legal documents that specify treatment preferences and surrogate decision-makers in the event someone becomes unable to make reasonable medical decisions on their own behalf. While advance directives have primarily been used for medical conditions such as if someone is incapacitated from a stroke, they are increasingly being used for psychiatric conditions that may also result in an individual lacking the capacity to make reasonable medical decisions for themselves.

Psychiatric advance directives are a great way to ensure someone's wishes are followed, even in instances when they may not be able to give reasonable medical consent, given time-limited psychiatric instability, and may decline care as a result, for example due to acute psychosis. In these instances, someone can specify what treatment they want and who they want to help them make medical or psychiatric decisions should they become unable to do so themselves.

There are three main types of advance directives: a living will, health care proxy, and durable power of attorney.

Living wills are legal documents that specify what types of medical treatment are desired, and can provide either general or very detailed instructions in specific situations. Living wills are most commonly used to address terminal and irreversible medical conditions; for example to request that interventions that prolong the dying process be withheld. In other instances, living wills provide more specific direction related to interventions such as the receipt of food or feeding tubes, intravenous fluids, antibiotics, breathing machines, or cardiopulmonary resuscitation (CPR).

Health care proxies are very relevant for psychiatric conditions, as they involve an individual with the condition designating another person to make health decisions on their behalf in the event they are unable to do so themselves. This is often a family member or trusted friend, and can be very useful in instances when loved ones may be acutely psychotic or manic and unable to make or communicate their own health decisions. In this way, health care proxies can empower individuals with serious mental illness to determine their care, even when their psychiatric condition precludes them from making reasonable health decisions on their own accord.

The last type of advance directive is a durable power of attorney, which is similar to health care proxies, except a durable power of attorney applies to designees that make financial and other decisions on the behalf of the impacted person in the event they are medically or psychiatrically unable to do so themselves. Whereas a health care proxy is designated to make health-related decisions for someone else, a durable power of attorney is designated to manage one's financial affairs.

While all types of advance directives can be helpful, for psychiatric conditions, health care proxies and durable power of attorney can be particularly useful and are increasingly common.

While hiring a lawyer to help with more complicated advance directives may cost several thousand dollars, more economical options are also available with online legal services or with free legal services that sometimes partner with behavioral health treatment programs.

In short, advance directives can provide extraordinary peace of mind, while also allowing space to have important conversations about how loved ones with serious mental illness would want their medical and potentially financial decisions handled, in the event their symptoms prevent them from making reasoned decisions.

Chapter Eight

Conclusion

Caregiving for someone with serious mental illness is often characterized by alternating periods of hope and progress, as well as the lowest of lows. Behavioral health systems can be extraordinarily convoluted and contribute to this rollercoaster. The various policy, clinical, legal, and practical considerations inherent in navigating these systems can challenge experts who work within the field, let alone families who are just finding out that their loved one may have a severe psychiatric condition that requires care.

Things were going great when I received a call from my mom in 2014. From the tone and hesitancy of her voice, I could tell that something was wrong. She said she felt a lump in her breast years ago and had only gone in to get it evaluated by a doctor when the pain became unbearable.

When my mom was first diagnosed with Stage IV breast cancer, I was prepared for challenges convincing her insurance to cover necessary care, uneasiness from her care team about sharing health information with family, and just generally feeling as if we were on our own regarding how to make sure that she received what she needed. Up to that point, I had only known what it was like to navigate behavioral health systems.

But after her cancer diagnosis, it became immediately clear that navigating the physical health system was going to be much different than our experiences seeking care for her schizophrenia. We were walked through needed documentation and phone calls to coordinate insurance and imaging appointments were made on our behalf.

When it came to my mom's breast cancer treatment, coordination with doctors was easy, and efforts were made to ensure family were informed of her care. This is opposed to how HIPAA is often twisted in mental health settings and cited as the reason for not sharing information with family. Whether due to genuine misunderstanding about HIPAA, implicit stigma and/or bias, or the fact that not sharing information generally requires less effort than sharing information, HIPAA was maneuvered around in physical health systems while it felt like it was hidden behind in mental health systems.

While navigating health systems for breast cancer treatment felt like a series of doors that others were helping us open, the voyage through mental health systems was like being dropped into a maze one had to stumble their way through.

For about three years, my mom responded well to her hormonal, non-chemo treatment. She experienced few side effects and, from the outside, it was difficult to even know that she was battling cancer. However, as is the unabating nature of cancer, it gradually evolves, often making impotent a previously effective treatment over time. Once the non-chemo treatment stopped working, we reluctantly moved on to the chemo options, which came with more side effects.

By the time my mom stopped responding to her breast cancer treatment altogether about five years after her diagnosis, we had numerous conversations about what was important to her, both in life and death.

Terminal cancer has an in-your-face way of reminding everyone just how finite life is, and of squeezing healthy and needed conversations out of even the most taciturn of individuals. We reminisced about family photos that we hadn't looked at in decades, and memories materialized in the world around us. We were able to say everything we needed and wanted to say, and most importantly, made crystal clear to Mom just how much she was loved, appreciated, and how much she would be missed. The hospice experience was simultaneously heartbreaking, draining, and precious.

After two devastatingly painful weeks, she was gone. My brother and I were holding her hand as she took her last breath.

Along the journey of my mom's life and death, we learned how love could make paranoia succumb to the more powerful need for connection between parent and child. And also, how it could hold families together and serve as a light through some of the deep, dark valleys of chronic schizophrenia. My personal and professional opinion as a psychiatrist is that ensuring that my mom felt unconditionally loved and cared for every step of the way was vital to her recovery; just as important as the medication prescribed to her and the therapy conducted by her care team.

Some final thoughts that would have been helpful for my family as we were undergoing our own journey navigating the behavioral health system:

You are not alone. There are many families going through something similar to what you're going through, including many families near you. The National Alliance on Mental Illness (NAMI; www.nami.org) organizes family support groups in most communities across the country and has a number of other helpful resources on their website.

The path to recovery is rarely linear, and both the journey and destination look different for everyone. You will be able to influence some aspects of your recovery journey and destination, while others will be out of your control. Recognizing what you can control and what you cannot, and when to push and when to pull back, is important to maintain one's stamina throughout this process. While empowering yourself with knowledge and resources/tools can maximize the influence you have on what happens as you seek care for your loved one, there will also inevitably be things outside of your control that you will need to recognize and accept in order to maintain your own well-being.

Compassionate advocacy from both the *inside* and the *outside* can be helpful. In this sense, compassionate advocacy refers to compassion for both who you are advocating for and who you are advocating to. There are many people (officials, administrators, practitioners, etc.) who want to do right by their constituents and clients, and are doing their best to help the very person or people you are wanting to help. Focusing advocacy on policies or issues is almost always more constructive and effective than focusing on people. While the *inside* refers to the immediate care team and practitioners associated with your loved one at a clinical and day-to-day level, the *outside* refers to extended circles of influencers such as local, state, or federal leadership that may be able to address systems- or policy-level barriers that can improve access and behavioral health care. Effective advocates know that *how* one approaches advocacy is just as important as *what* they are advocating for.

Self-care and caring for others are not mutually exclusive, so it is essential to remember to also take care of yourself. The path to accessing behavioral health care is unfortunately often more challenging than it should be, given various community-level, policy-level, and clinical-level opportunities and challenges related to navigating behavioral health systems. While we advocate for compassion for people living with behavioral health conditions, it is also important that caregivers have compassion for themselves as well. It is okay to take time for yourself and to nourish your own well-being as you also seek the well-being of those you're caring for.

Hopefully, this book has helped to establish a framework for better understanding serious mental illness and the intricacies of behavioral health systems, as well as the knowledge and tools needed to successfully navigate behavioral health systems and make the journey a bit easier.

Made in the USA
Middletown, DE
22 July 2022